SOMATIC YOGA

28-Day Plan to Release Stress and Anxiety with Low-Impact Exercises | Quick & Easy Routines to Lose Weight - Video Guide Included

Jane Hum

DISCLAIMER

The information provided in this book is intended for educational and informational purposes only. It is not a substitute for professional medical advice, diagnosis, or treatment. Always seek the advice of your physician or other qualified healthcare provider before starting any new fitness program or making any changes to an existing one. The author and publisher of this book are not responsible for any injury or health problems that may result from the use of the information in this book.

TABLE OF CONTENTS

INTRODUCTION

Hello! I'm sure this book will serve as a helpful guide for enhancing both your physical and mental well-being. I really hope this book exceeds your expectations!

Somatic exercises offer numerous benefits, including trauma release, increased flexibility, a strengthened mind-body connection, stress relief, a deeper connection with your body, and hormone regulation (vital for weight loss and body recomposition). These practices emphasize the interconnectedness of body, mind, and spirit, and they extend beyond mere physical activity to embody a comprehensive approach to health. They can also drastically help in weight loss and provide additional advantages.

Within this book you will find:

- *A special section that addresses common questions about somatic exercises*, including their benefits, essential information, tips to stay motivated long-term, and the best ways to engage with the exercises.
- *More than 30 selected exercises designed to enhance your well-being* and happiness like never before. Each exercise is a step towards becoming the best version of yourself to unlock your body's full potential and achieve tranquility.
- *A 28-day plan with easy-to-follow routines* to guide your daily progress. This structured approach keeps you motivated and on course, as you start your journey with somatic practices.
- And there's more – *you'll find plenty of insightful information, tips, and inspiration throughout this book*. Prepare to explore, learn, and feel the transformative effects of somatic exercises on your life!

Also, for any questions or doubts about the exercises and the training plan, feel free to email me at somatictrainingplan@gmail.com

4 SIMPLE & EFFECTIVE TIPS TO KEEP YOUR MOTIVATION HIGH

Here are some simple tips to help you stick with your 28-day exercise plan:

Find an Accountability Partner

It's more fun to do things with a friend! If you both do the exercises together, it can help you keep going, even on days when you might not feel like it.

Picture Your Success

Think about how awesome you'll look and feel at the end of the 28 days. Maybe you'll feel stronger or simply better overall. Keep that picture in your mind to help you keep exercising, even when it's tough.

Remember Why You Started

Sometimes, you might not want to exercise because you're too busy or just tired. When that happens, try to remember why you started. Maybe you wanted to be stronger or just feel better. Write this down and look at it when you need a little push.

Write it Down

After you exercise, write down how you feel. Were you happy? Tired? A little sore? Writing it down will help you see how much you've improved by the end of the 28 days, which is really cool!

20 COMMON QUESTIONS ABOUT SOMATIC EXERCISES

1. What are somatic exercises?

Somatic exercises, developed in the 1970s, focus on healing from trauma, reducing stress, and enhancing physical well-being through mindful, sensory movements that emphasize the mind-body connection as well as enhancing weight loss.

2. How long are the sessions?

Typically, sessions range from 10 to 20 minutes. Consistency is crucial to get the most out of it - the 28-day plan is designed to keep you motivated during the whole training with a variety of exercises.

3. Why choose somatic exercises?

This method is particularly effective for enhancing mental and spiritual well-being through physical movement, making it ideal for those seeking stress reduction and overall physical improvement.

4. What are the benefits?

These exercises offer physical, mental, and spiritual gains, such as increased flexibility, calorie burn, stress and anxiety relief, trauma healing, and a stronger connection with your body.

5. What is the best way to read the book?

Understand the structure of the book, which includes exercise explanations followed by a 28-day plan with a routine. Ideally, review the exercises daily before starting.

6. How to read the book with images and explanations?

First, look at the images to understand the exercises visually, then read the detailed explanations to perform the exercises correctly.

7. Why are somatic exercises effective for weight loss?

They help manage stress and trauma, which can reduce stress-induced overeating and sedentary behaviors. They also promote a cycle of well-being through regular physical activity and improved mental health.

8. Best time of day for the exercises?

This varies by individual preference; some find morning sessions energizing, while others prefer evening sessions to unwind.

9. What to do after the 28-day plan?

Take a short break, then repeat part of the program with increased intensity to continue improving. More details about what to do are provided at the end of the 28-day plan, on page 82. If you have any doubts, feel free to email me at somatictrainingplan@gmail.com.

10. Effect of two workouts a day?

Stick to the planned single daily session for maximum benefit, as doubling up does not accelerate benefits and may lead to burnout.

11. Who can do somatic exercises?

Anyone looking to improve mental health, physical condition, or recover from trauma can benefit from these exercises. Any level is welcomed. The exercises have a section called "Note", where you can find tips on how to make the exercises more challenging (where necessary).

12. Are somatic exercises useful for trauma healing?

Yes, they are designed to help release physical tension associated with trauma, incorporating techniques that enhance relaxation and body awareness.

13. How do I know if I am releasing trauma?

Trauma release can manifest in various physical and emotional reactions, such as crying or laughing, typically occurring naturally over time.

14. What if I feel nausea during the exercises?

Avoid eating heavily before exercising, adjust the intensity as needed, and consult a healthcare professional if discomfort continues. These exercises should make you feel better, not worse.

15. Is walking a somatic exercise?

Mindful walking, or "Walking Meditation," is considered part of somatic practices, emphasizing body and movement awareness. It is especially true when you walk without electronics to keep you engaged in something other than walking.

16. Is meditation a somatic exercise?

Meditation complements somatic exercises by fostering mindfulness and stress relief, although it's more focused on mental rather than physical activity.

17. Do somatic exercises improve mood?

Yes, they improve mood by enhancing physical fitness, alleviating pain, and triggering the release of mood-regulating neurotransmitters like dopamine.

18. What does the mind-body connection mean?

Developing a mind-body connection involves becoming attuned to your body's signals and tensions, which is vital for recognizing and addressing areas where trauma is held.

19. What to focus on during the exercises?

Concentrate on your breathing and the sensations in your body, allowing thoughts to pass without engaging with them to enhance the effectiveness of the practice. In the exercises, I will mention what to focus on, so no worries...I got you covered!

20. What positive changes can I expect after finishing the book?

Expect reduced stress, enhanced mood, weight loss, better fitness, trauma healing, and a deeper understanding of your body and its needs.

SOMATIC EXERCISES

CIRCLING HIPS

Here's a simple exercise to help loosen up tight hips and help manage your stress levels

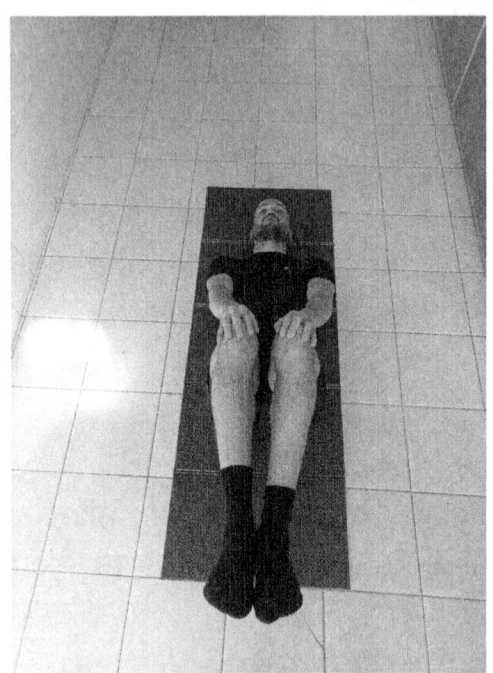

Step 1 - *Starting position.*

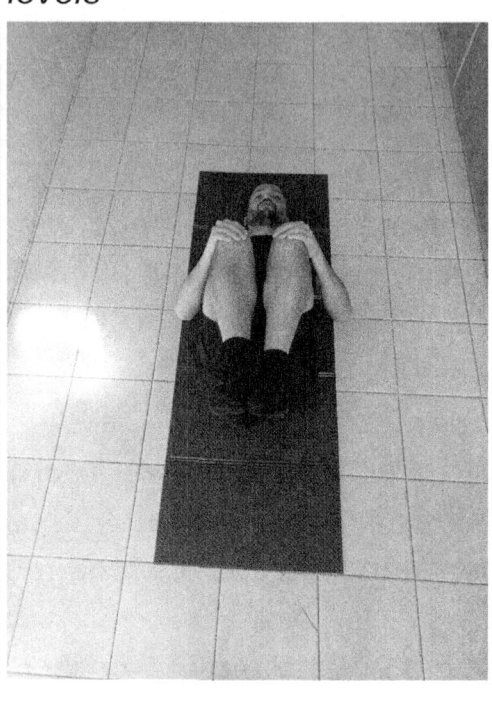

Step 2 - *Knees towards your chest.*

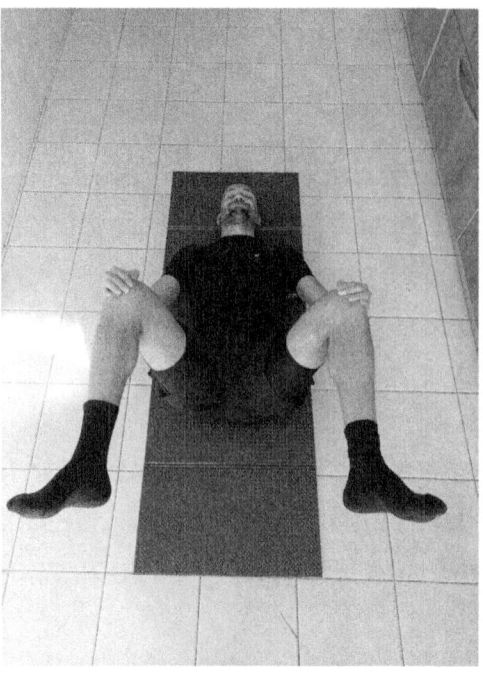

Step 3 - *Draw circles with your knees.*

How to Do it:

1. Begin by lying down on a mat. Bend your knees so your feet are off the floor and place your hands on your knees. Take slow, deep breaths to relax.
2. Then, gently pull your knees toward your chest, keeping them close together. This also helps stretch the lower back and hips.
3. Next, slowly open your knees out to the sides as wide as comfortable, then bring them back together. Imagine you are drawing a circle with your knees. This movement helps loosen the hip joints.
4. Do this movement for the number of repetitions mentioned. Make sure to move slowly and breathe normally as you perform the circles.

Note:

The first time you do this exercise, you might feel a little nauseous as your muscles release tension that has built up over the years. To help prevent nausea, drink plenty of water before and after your workout. This will keep you hydrated and help flush out any released toxins.

Also, as a beginner as you bring your knees toward your chest, it's very common to accidentally hold your breath, which isn't helpful. Instead, make sure to exhale fully as you pull your knees in. This will help you relax deeper into the position. Keep your breathing steady and deep throughout the exercise to help your body relax and maximize the stretch in your hips.

If you have any issues downloading the QR code or if it does not open, please email me at somatictrainingplan@gmail.com, and I will assist you.

ROBOT SIDE-TO-SIDE

This exercise is excellent for easing neck and shoulder tension, improving posture, and strengthening your core.

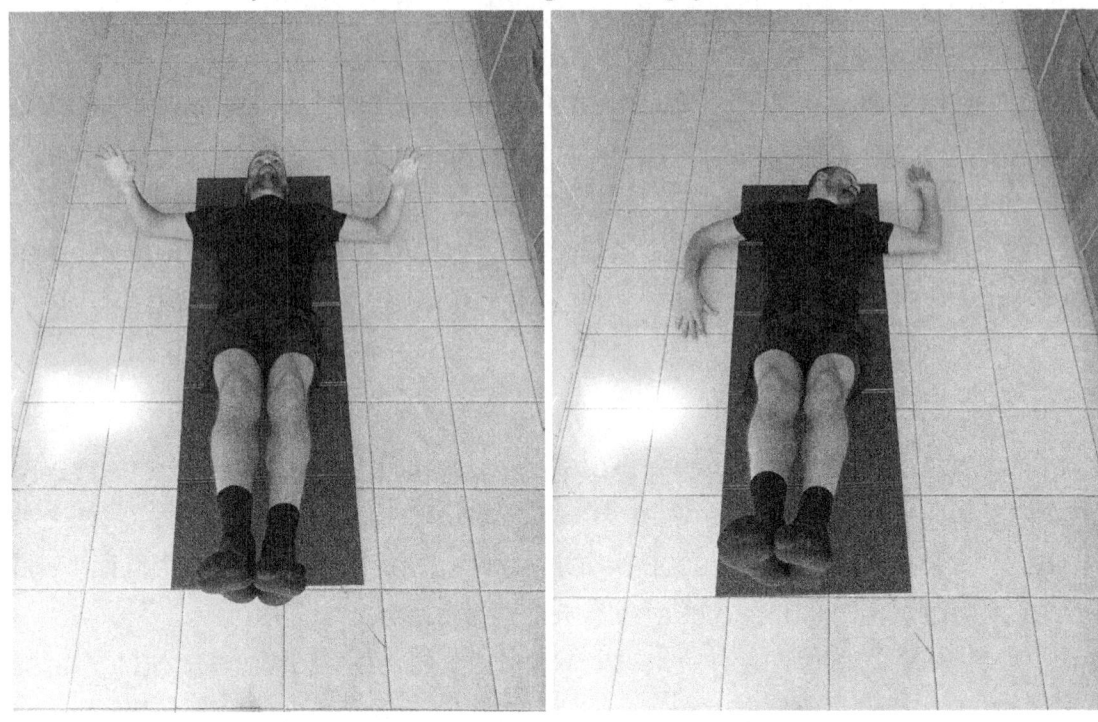

Step 1 - *Lift your legs and forearms.*   **Step 2** - *Lower your forearms and turn your head.*

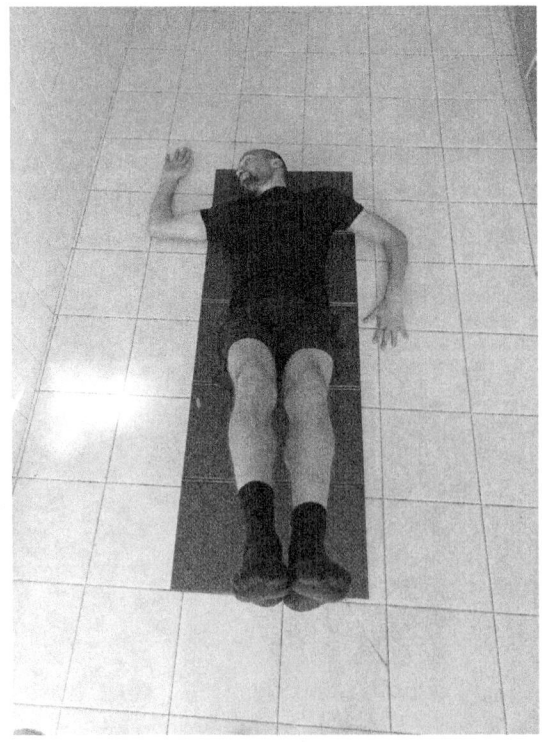

Step 3 - Then, repeat on the other side.

How to Do it:

1. Begin by lying on your back and raising your legs as shown. Keep your arms stretched out to the sides with your forearms lifted. This is the starting position.
2. Next, lower your left forearm to the floor with your left hand pointing over your head, while your right forearm goes to the floor with your hand pointing down toward your feet. At the same time, turn your head toward your left hand - see image 2. Exhale deeply once you get to this position.
3. After that, return to the starting position, and then repeat the same movement on the other side.
4. Perform the mentioned reps, alternating sides.

Note:

This exercise not only works your core but also helps improve your posture in a unique way. If it's too hard, you can start by keeping your legs on the floor. When you're ready, try the full exercise as shown in the pictures.

Every time you rotate your head remember to breathe out and release all the tension accumulated.

ADVANCED CRAWLING

This exercise is fantastic for building strength in your lower body and core, while also enhancing coordination with your body.

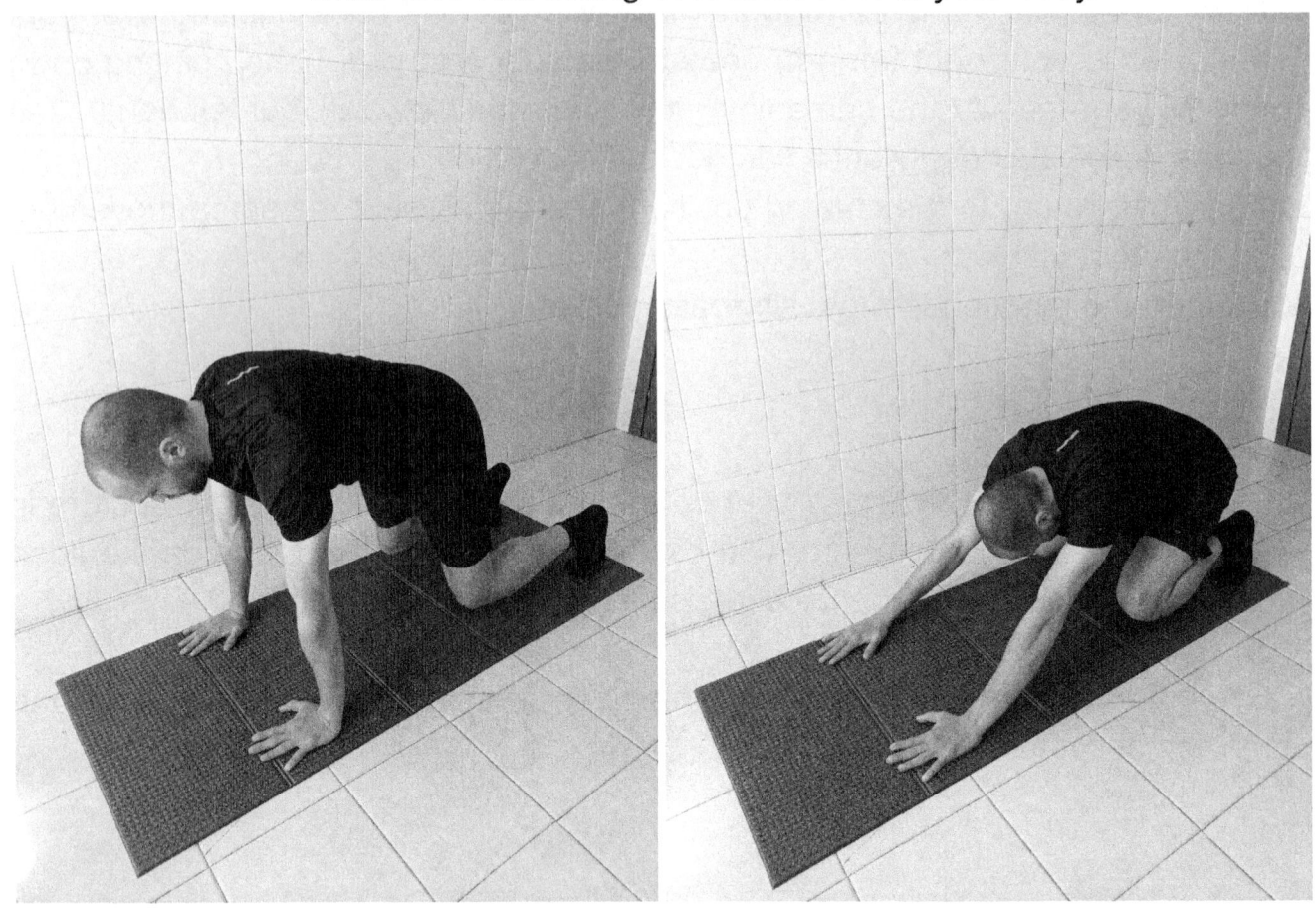

Step 1 - *Start on hands and feet with knees slightly lifted.*   **Step 2** - *Final position: stretching your back.*

How to Do it:

1. Place your hands on the mat with your arms straight and your shoulders directly above your hands. Bend your knees to engage your quadriceps, and lift them off the mat so only your toes and hands are touching. Hold this position for 1 second and breathe in through your nose.
2. Next, slowly bring your hips closer to your heels to stretch your back while keeping your knees elevated and your arms straight, as shown in the second image. Breathe out, and hold this position for one second.
3. Lastly, come back to the starting position and repeat the exercise for the mentioned reps.

Note:

Perform the exercise slowly and with control, focusing on your body's movements. It requires both strength and balance. Breathe out deeply through your mouth to release any tension and bring yourself into the present moment.

SEATED UPPER TWIST

Great exercise to release tension in your trunk mobilizing your spine.

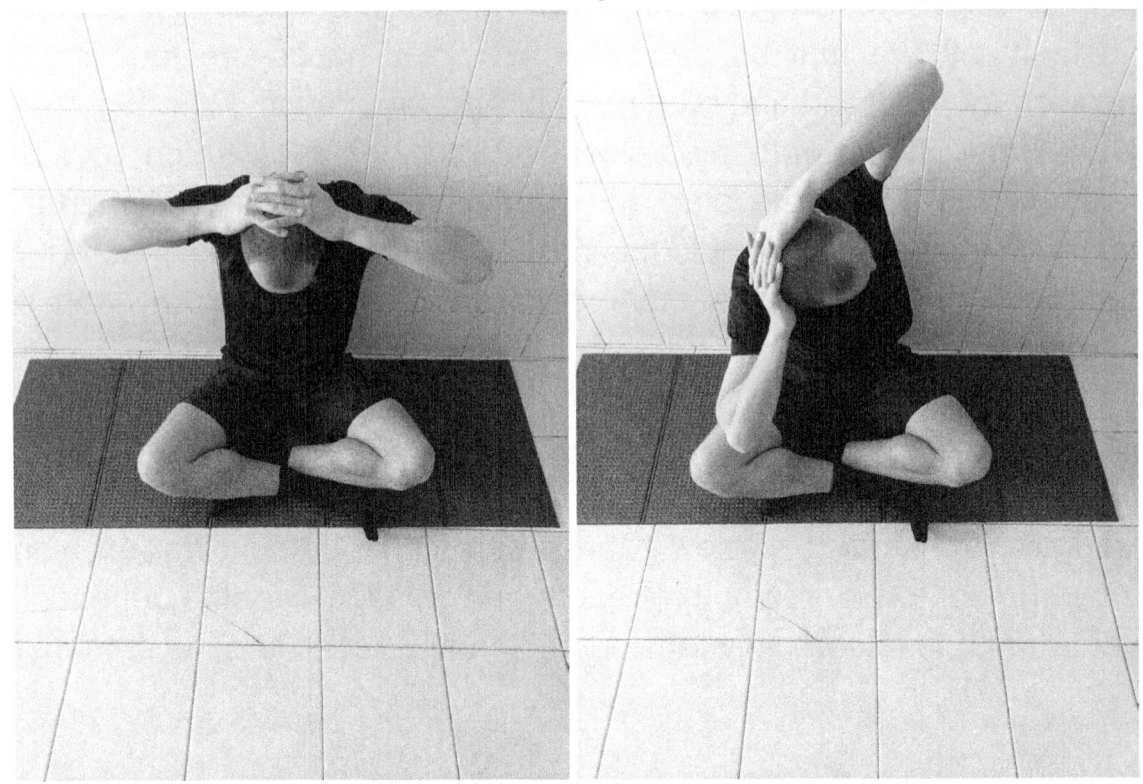

Step 1 - *Starting position with legs crossed.*   **Step 2** - *Rotate towards the left side.*

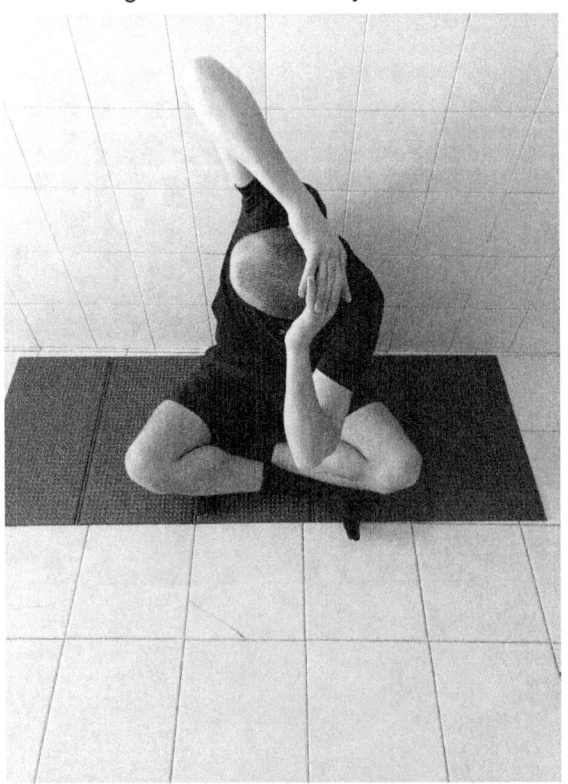

Step 3 - *Then, repeat on the other side.*

How to Do it:

1. To start, sit on the mat with your legs crossed and your back straight. Put both hands on the back of your head, as illustrated in the first image.
2. Next, gently lower your head until your chin nearly touches your collarbone. Adjust until you find a comfortable position.
3. Gradually, while keeping your hands on the back of your head, turn your face to the left as you breathe out. You'll feel a stretch in your sides and neck. Check the second image for guidance.
4. Return to the starting position while inhaling.
5. Then, repeat it on the other side. One rep is now complete.
6. Repeat it for the mentioned reps.

Note:

This exercise is excellent for releasing feelings of distress and discouragement that often build up in the neck and upper body, affecting posture and flexibility. If these feelings and tightness aren't released, they can lead to stress and pain. Plus, this position is beneficial for knee health.

LUNGE RELAXATION

This exercise is fantastic for building strength in your lower body, improving your mind-body connection, and enhancing coordination.

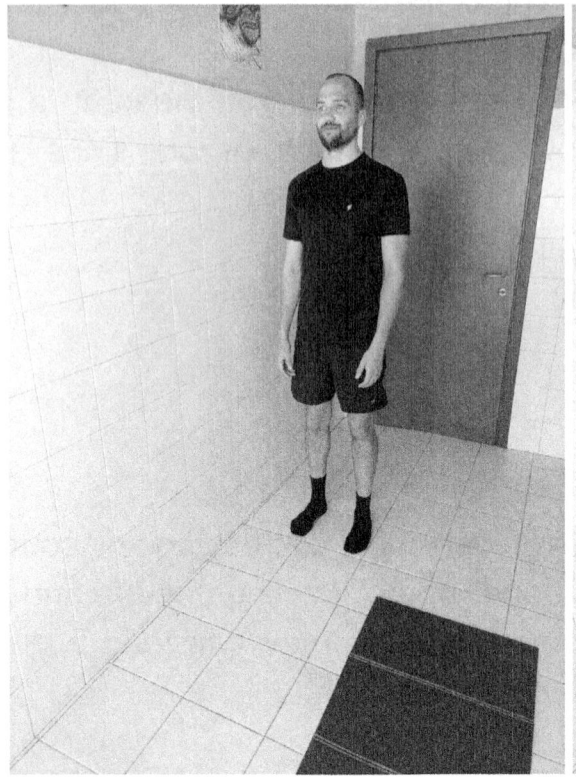

Step 1 *- Starting position.*

Step 2 *- Lunge with your right leg.*

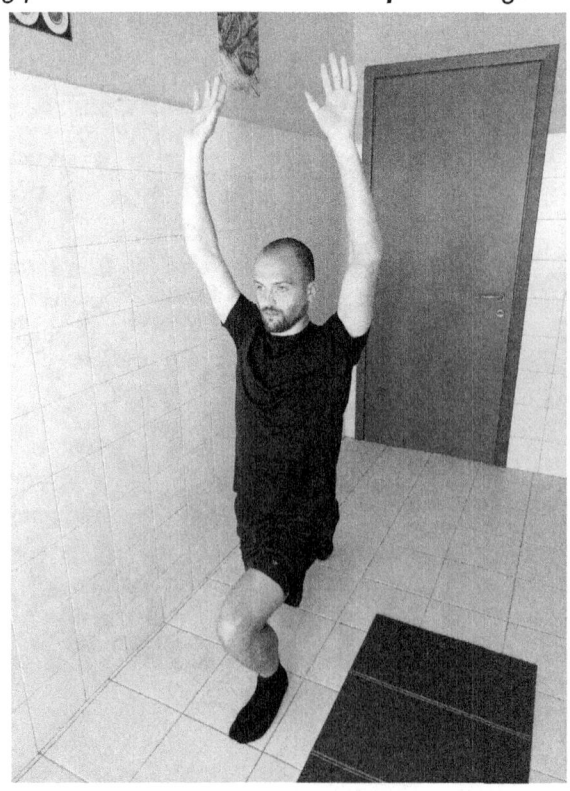

Step 3 *- Then, repeat with the left leg.*

How to Do it:

1. Stand with your feet hip-width apart and your arms at your sides. Take a deep breath in through your nose, noticing how your body feels.
2. Next, step forward into a lunge with your right leg. Try to get your right thigh parallel to the floor and your left knee close to the ground. As you do this, extend your arms over your head and exhale completely.
3. Then, return to the starting position and repeat the same movement on your left side. Keep alternating sides for the number of repetitions mentioned.

Note:

If you're struggling with balance, try focusing on a specific point a few feet away. This can help you stay stable. Also, remember to inhale as you return to the starting position. Concentrate on releasing all tension as you lunge and inhale all the energy around you as you come back to the starting position.

If you have any issues downloading the QR code or if it does not open, please email me at somatictrainingplan@gmail.com, and I will assist you.

STANDING KNEE UP

This exercise is fantastic for improving your balance and coordination, and it also helps make your lower body more flexible. The "hugging" part can make you feel happier and more positive.

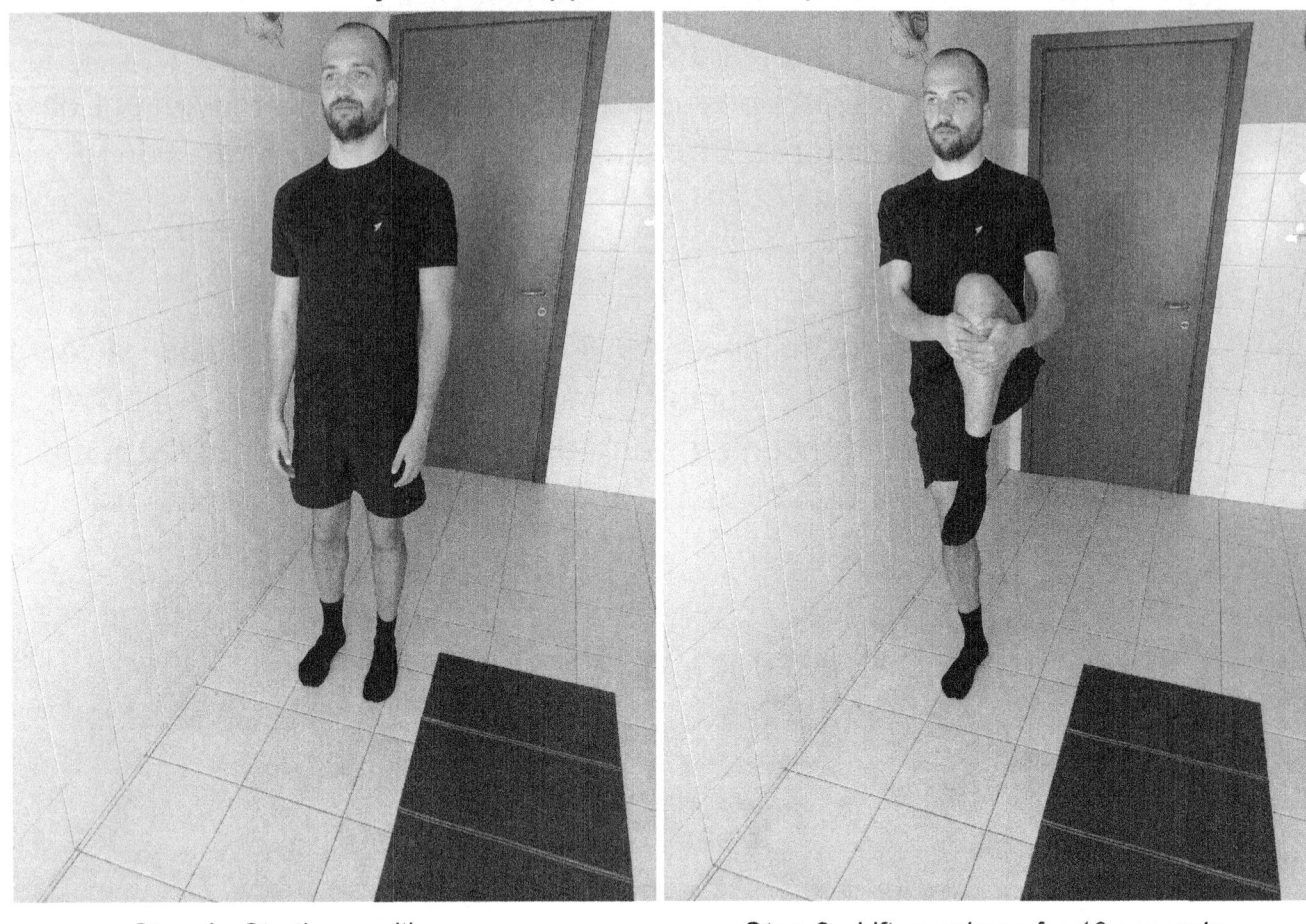

Step 1 - *Starting position.*   **Step 2** - *Lift your knee for 10 seconds.*

If you have any questions or doubts, feel free to contact me at somatictrainingplan@gmail.com and I'll be happy to assist you the best I can about somatic exercises and workouts!

How to Do it:

1. Start by standing on the mat with your arms next to your body. Take a gentle breath in.
2. Next, using both hands, bring one knee close to your chest while keeping only one foot on the floor. Focus on breathing deeply and slowly, inhaling through your nose and exhaling through your mouth.
3. Stay in this position for 10 seconds, breathing gently the whole time.
4. Afterward, return to the starting position, and then repeat the same movement on the other leg. Keep alternating sides for the number of repetitions mentioned.

Note:

If you're having trouble with balance, try focusing on a specific point on the floor a few feet away. Staring at something can help you feel steadier.

Also, if holding for 10 seconds feels too hard, try doing each position for 5 seconds instead. Eventually, as you practice, your balance will get better, and you'll manage to hold each position for 10 seconds easily.

ADVANCED BODY CIRCLES

This is a fantastic exercise to mobilize your spine and be confident in your body.

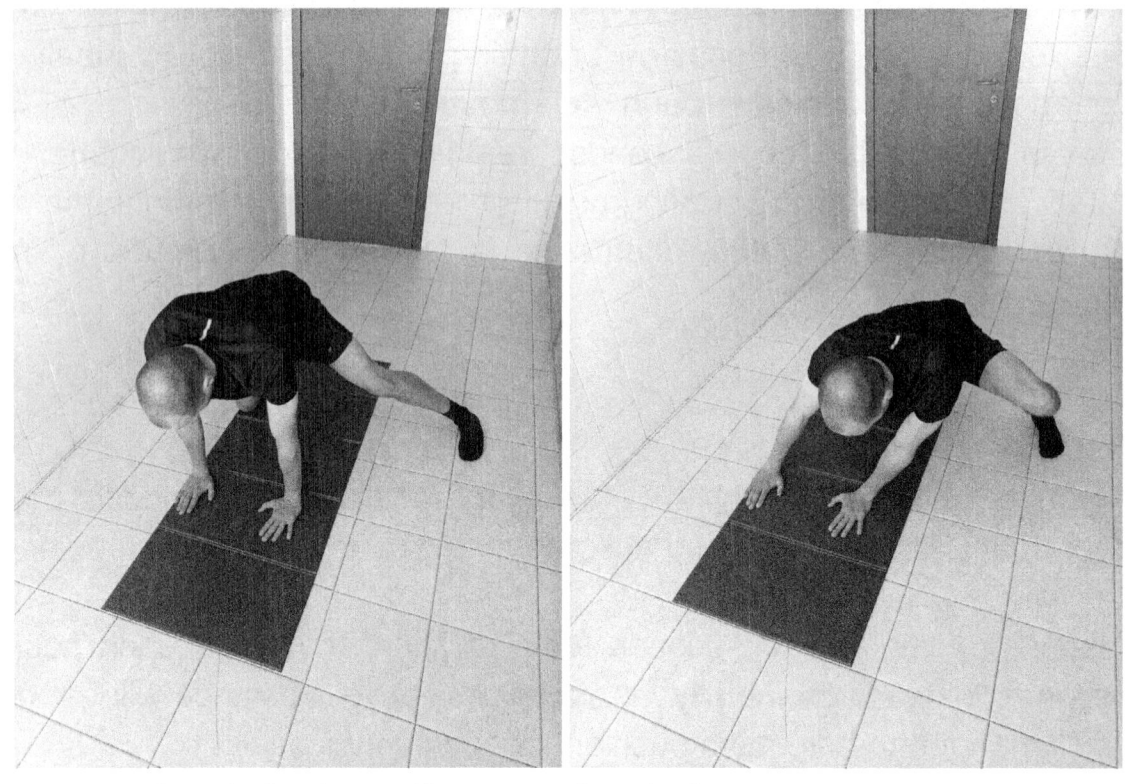

Step 1 - Starting position.   *Step 2 - Start moving your hips to the side.*

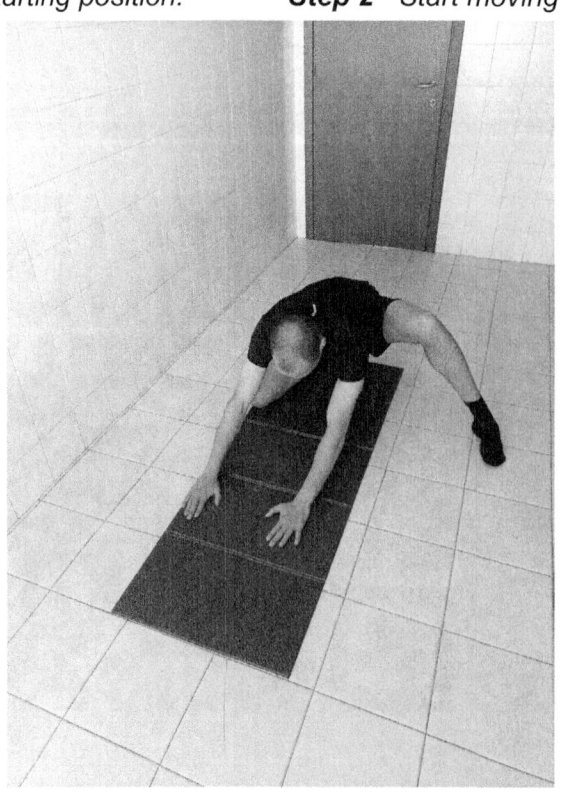

Step 3 - Then, move them backwards and repeat the motion as mentioned.

How to Do it:

1. Start placing the right shin on the floor while the left leg opens up to the side with your foot on the floor. The hands are in contact with the floor, just in front of you - see image.
2. From there simply move your hips and trunk in a circular way exploring new ranges of motion. Do the movement slowly and controlled
3. Repeat for the mentioned reps and then switch sides.

Note:

Make sure not to tense your muscles, but to stay loose and breathe softly, inhaling through your nose and exhaling through your mouth during the execution.

DIAGONAL OPENED TWIST

Great exercise to open up your upper body area that due to modern lifestyle tends to be quite stiff and closed up.

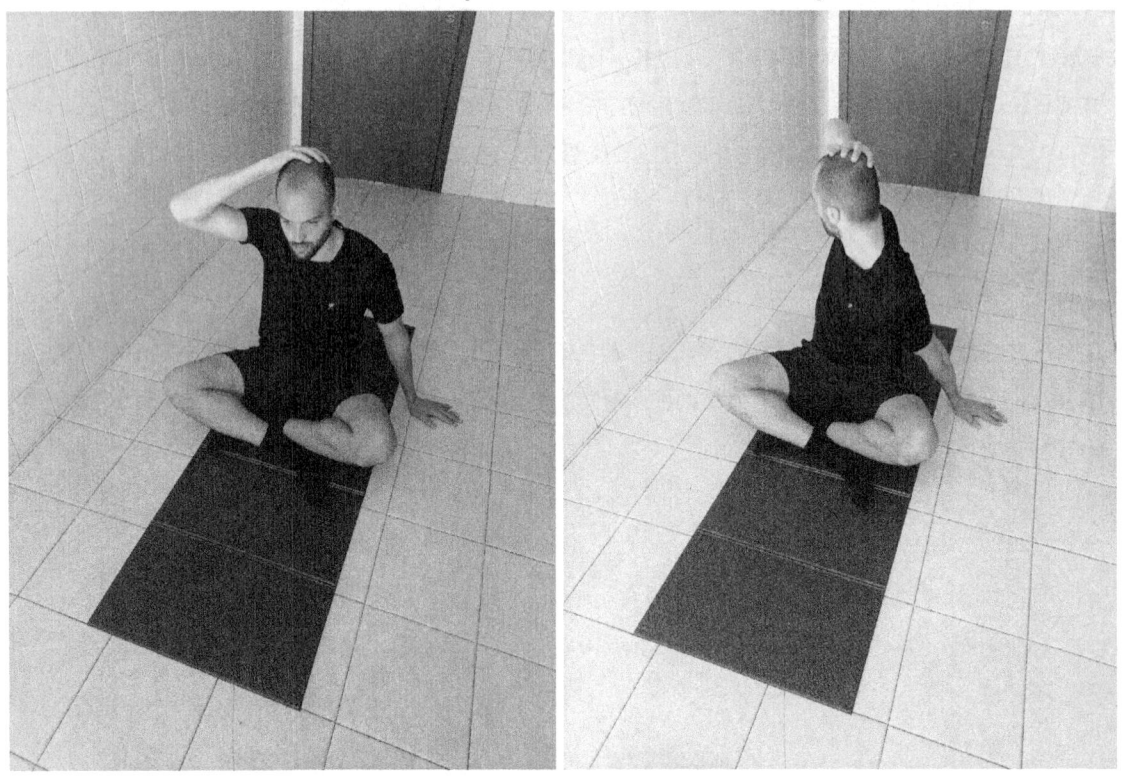

Step 1 *- Starting position.*   ***Step 2*** *- Open up your shoulder.*

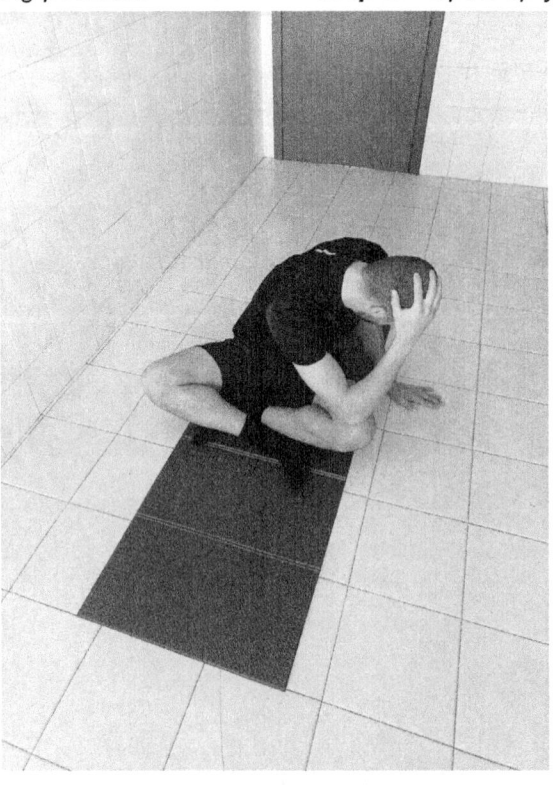

Step 3 *- Then, close your right elbows towards your left knee.*

How to Do it:

1. Begin by sitting with your legs crossed. Take a deep breath and place your right hand behind your head.
2. From there open up your body towards the right side. Look behind you. Keep the position for 2 seconds exhaling completely, and then come back into the starting position.
3. Then, try to reach with your right elbow towards your left knee. Do it slowly.
4. Then, come back into a seated position with your back straight. Inhale through your nose as you do so.
5. Repeat for the mentioned reps
6. Lastly, perform it on the other side.

Note:

When you do the second part of the movement there is no need to go all the way down to your knee if that seems too much for you. Do your best to perform this movement without exaggerating.

SUPINE STRETCH AND TWIST

It improves balance, flexibility, and relieves lower back pain, as well as reducing tension in your hip and shoulder area.

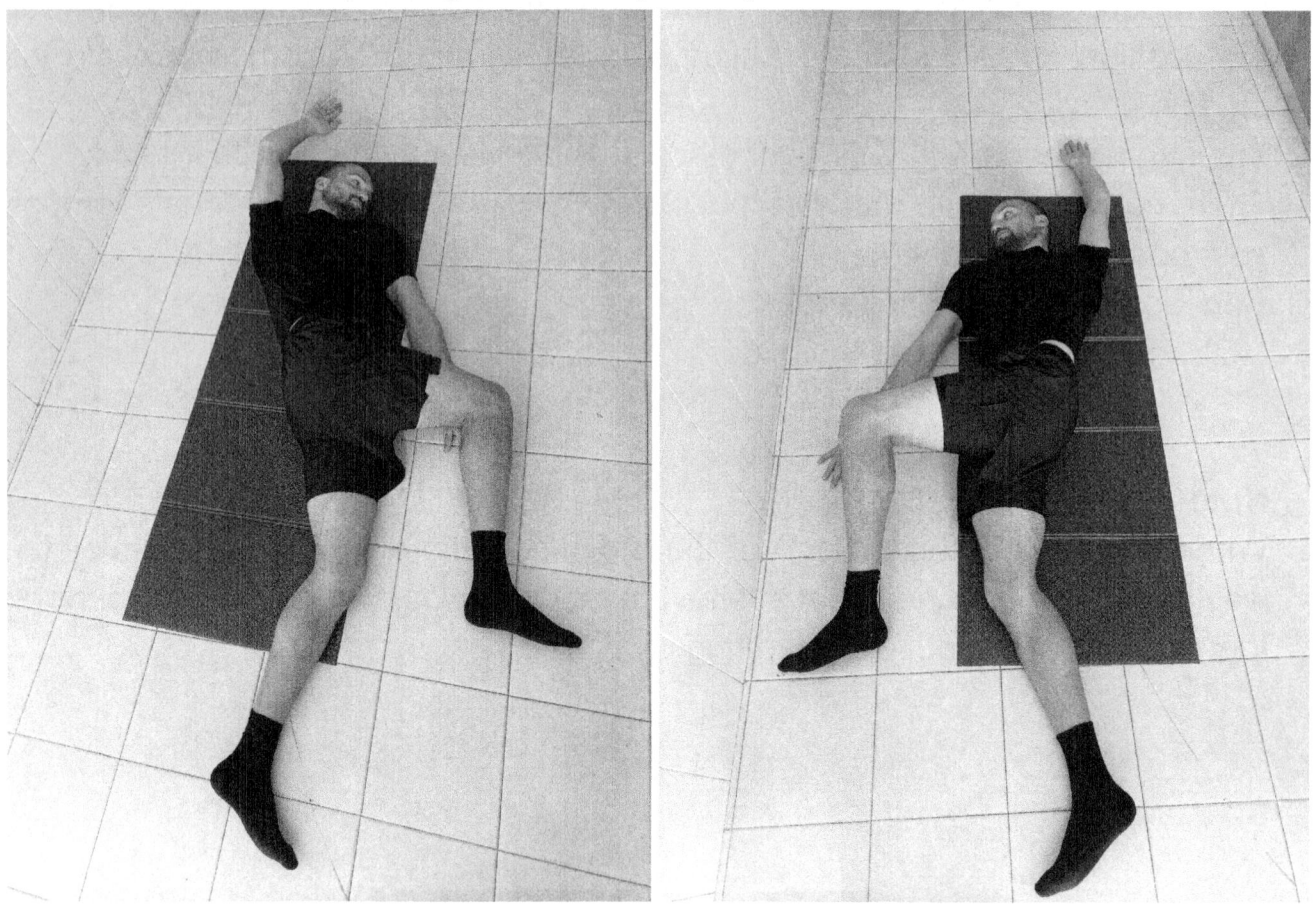

Step 1 - *Rotate towards the left and stretch.*   **Step 2** - *Repeat on the other side.*

How to Do it:

1. Lie on your back and bring the right leg over to the other side. By doing that you'll feel a mild stretch on your hips area as you are twisting your torso on one side - Turn your head towards the left side as you do so whilst keeping the right shoulder on the mat (see image and video for further assistance).
2. Then, bring your right arm over the head, aiming to stretch the side of your back gently.
3. Hold this position for a few breaths (2 to 4 breaths works well), imagining after each exhale that your body gets heavier and sinks down.
4. Then, perform one rep (a few breaths) on the other side.
5. Keep alternating the reps between the sides, as mentioned in the training plan.

Note:

This is a great exercise to release all the tension accumulated. It is great to have such exercises mixed with more intense ones because you always have to be able to wind down as you wish, even when you're sweating.

This is going to translate in real life, with you being able to face challenges and traumas and quickly shift into a more calm and centered version of yourself.

If you have any issues downloading the QR code or if it does not open, please email me at somatictrainingplan@gmail.com, and I will assist you.

SHOULDER OPENING

Here's a simple exercise to help calm feelings of anxiety

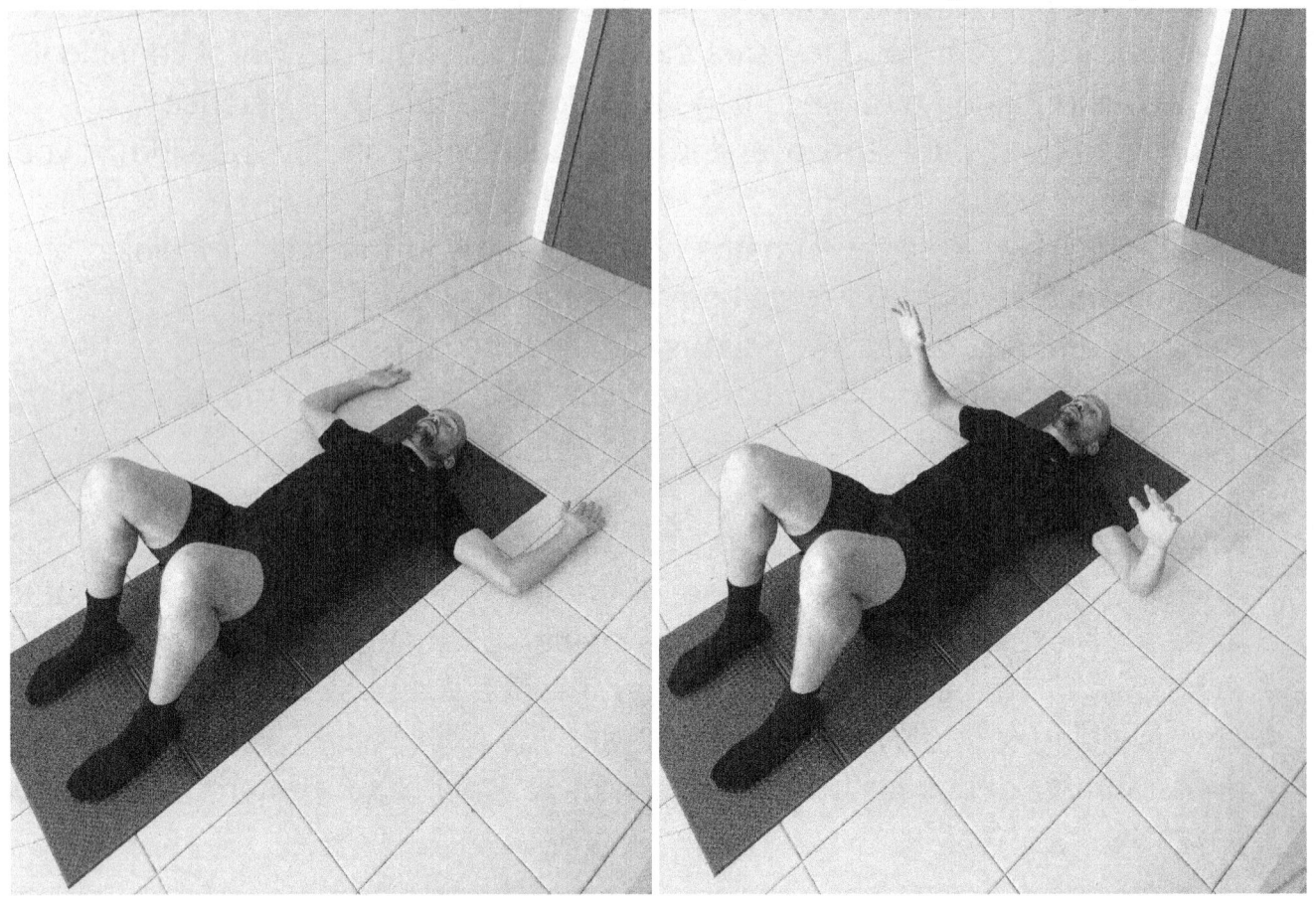

Step 1 - Starting position.   *Step 2 - Lift your forearms and inhale as you do so.*

How to Do it:

1. Begin by lying on your back on the floor. Bend your knees so that your feet are flat on the floor, and place your arms at a 90-degree angle with your forearms resting on the floor.
2. While breathing out gently, lift your forearms so they are pointing straight up to the ceiling. Hold this position for 1 second.
3. Slowly move your arms back to the starting position while breathing in through your nose.
4. Do this movement for the number of times mentioned.

Note:

The key to this exercise is to move smoothly to help loosen up the upper back and shoulder area, where we often hold a lot of stress and unprocessed feelings. This can make you feel more relaxed and less anxious.

SEATED CHAIR TWIST

Perfect exercise to both increase your heart rate & work on your full body movement + make sure to be in line with your breathing releasing all the tension accumulated.

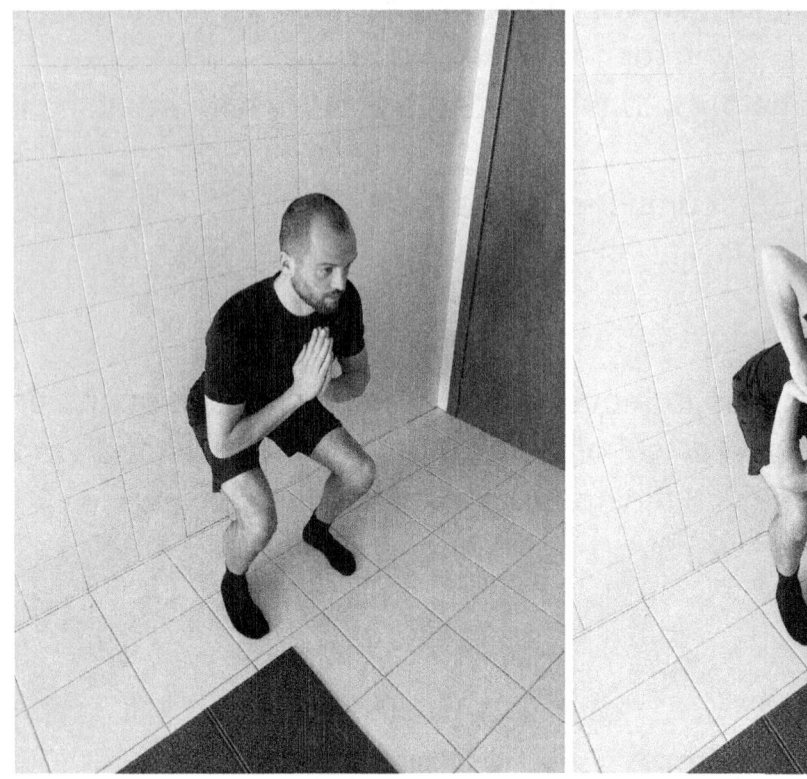

Step 1- *Starting position.*   **Step 2-** *Rotate your trunk to the side.*

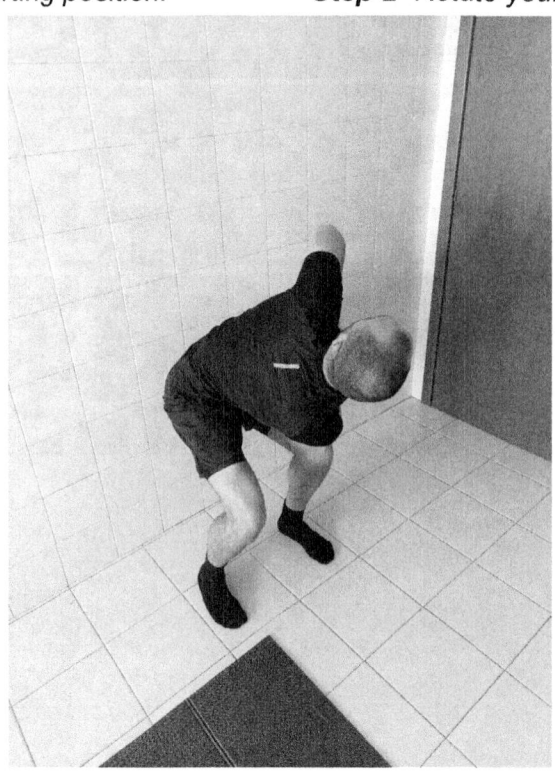

Step 3 - *Then, repeat on the other side.*

How to Do it:

1. Start in a standing position with your hands together at chest height and your feet slightly wider than hip-width apart.
2. From there, squat down (inhale gently as you do so).
3. Then, twist on one side, placing the opposite elbow down to the thigh. Look up towards the ceiling and breathe. Keep this position for 2 seconds.
4. Then, while keeping a squat position, switch to the other side.
5. Repeat for the mentioned reps, alternating the sides.

Note:

To make it more challenging in terms of strength and flexibility, it is suggested to bring your thighs almost parallel to the floor. Holding this position will require a good level of strength, balance, and flexibility.

To make it easier, do not go down as much, performing a squat that is easier on your legs.

RIVER STRETCH

This exercise aims at enhancing balance and flexibility as well as working on the side of your trunk.

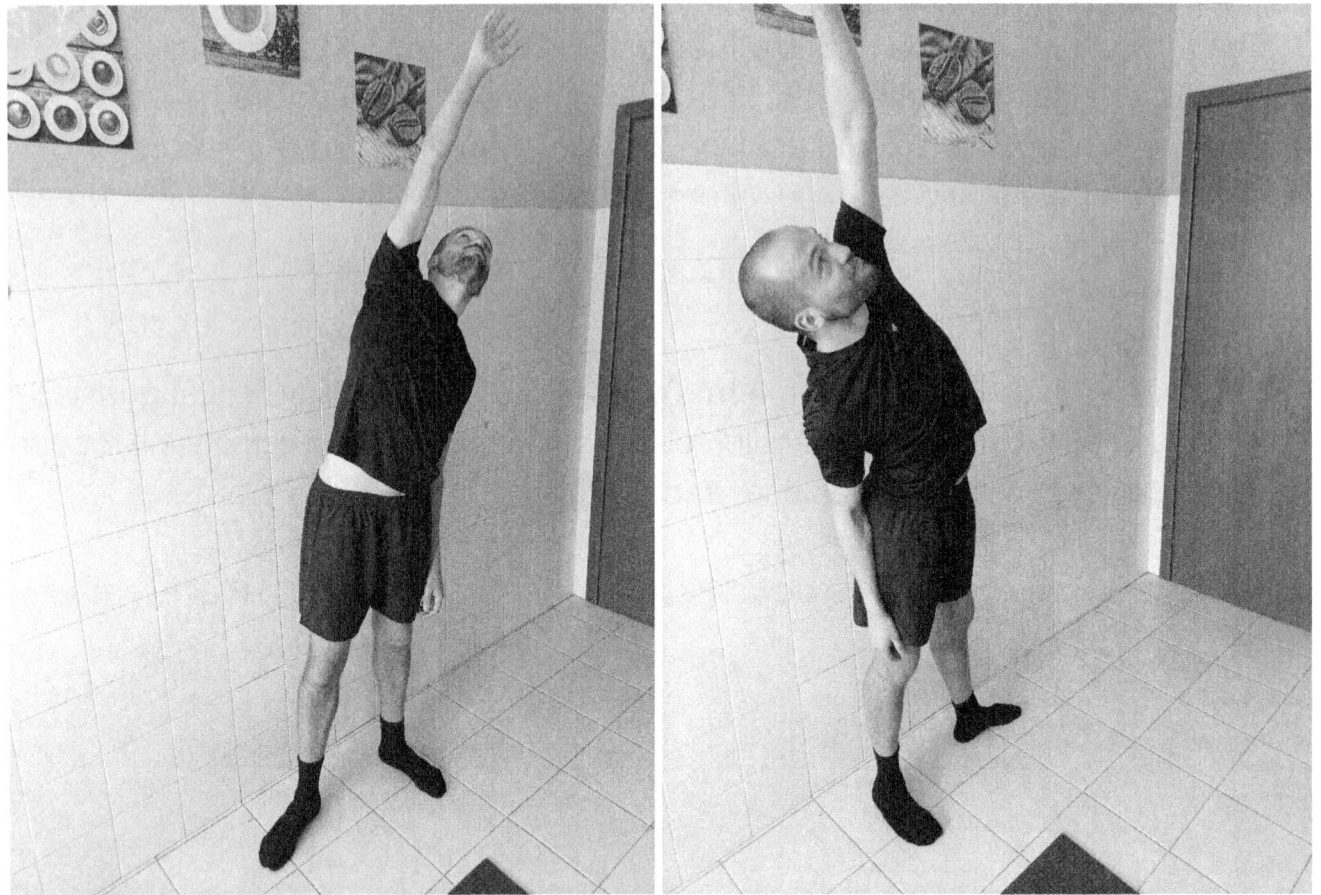

Step 1 - *Stretch on one side.*   **Step 2** - *Then, stretch the other side.*

How to Do it:

1. Begin by standing with your feet wider than hip-width apart and the right foot pointing out to the side.
2. The left arm is on the side of your body whilst your right arm reaches over your head, stretching it as much as you can - Look up to the ceiling.
3. Hold this position for 2 seconds, exhale deeply and then come back to the starting position, and repeat for the mentioned reps.
4. Lastly, repeat on the other side.

Note:

Perform this movement slowly and with control, as doing it too quickly might cause you to lose balance and/or not fully experience the benefits of stretching your upper body as intended by this exercise.

PEAK TOE PULSES

This exercise is fantastic for connecting with your body, releasing emotional tension, and enhancing mobility through simple movements.

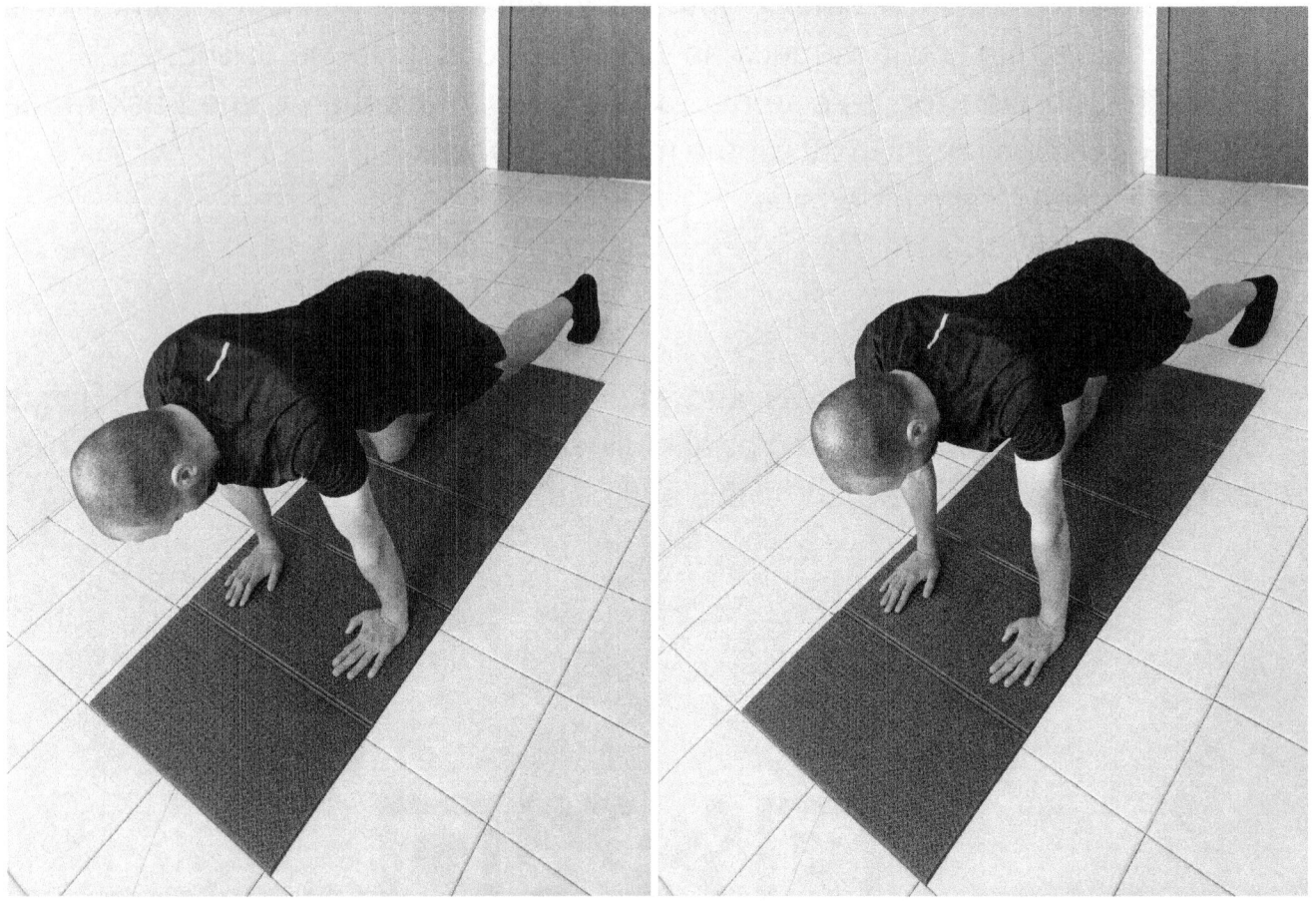

Step 1 - *Starting position*

Step 2 - *Swing gently hips for the specified time (see video).*

How to Do it:

1. Begin in a half-plank position, with your arms straight. Hands, right knee, and left foot on the floor. Check the first image for more guidance.
2. From there, shift your hips slightly back, as shown in the image, while bringing the left heel as close as possible to the ground.
3. Next, swiftly pulse with your toes and move forward, perform this movement smoothly.
4. Continue repeating this sequence for the specified number of seconds. Then, switch sides and repeat the exercise on the other side.

Note:

Make sure to keep breathing steadily and avoid holding your breath while performing this movement. Inhale and exhale as you move through the exercise. It is suggested to scan the QR Code below to ensure you're doing it correctly.

ACTIVE PIGEON STRETCH

This is a great exercise to enhance coordination, body control, and posture as well as releasing tension in the hips and back area.

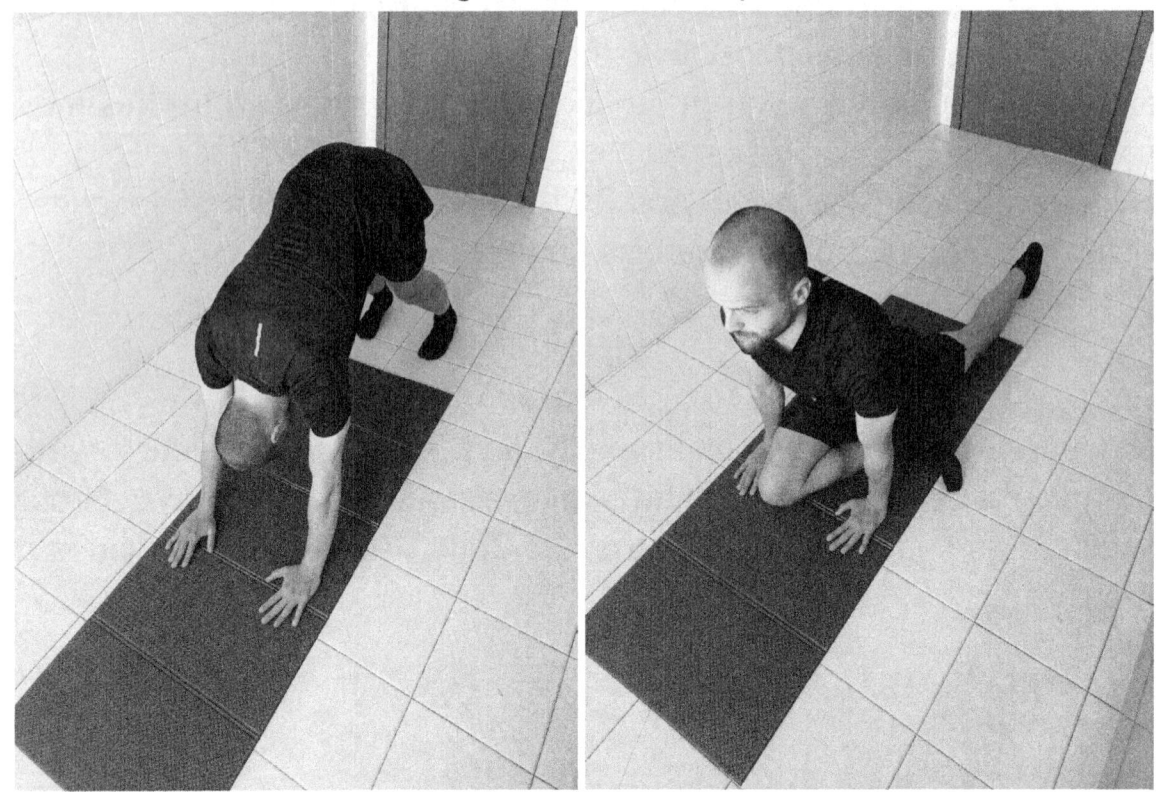

Step 1 - *Lift your glutes up.*   **Step 2** - *Draw your right knee between your legs, chest up.*

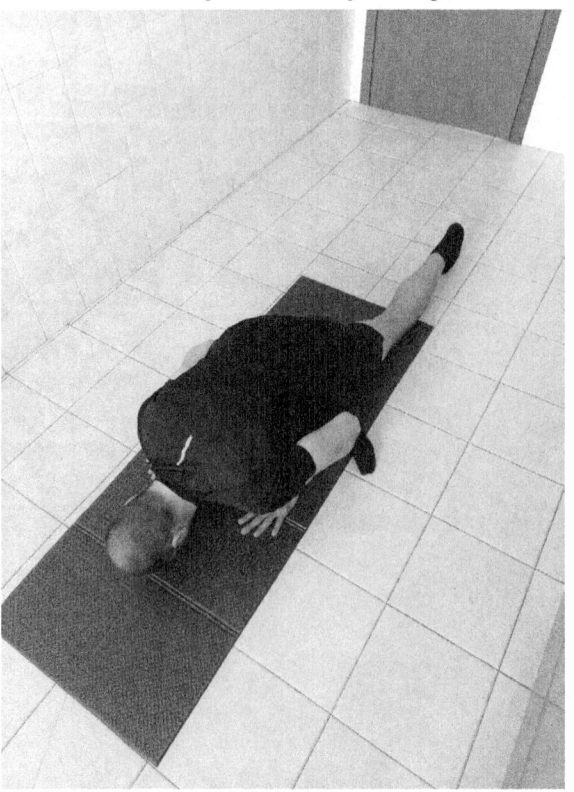

Step 3 - *Bring your chest as close as possible to the mat to feel a deeper stretch - breathe deeply.*

How to Do it:

1. Start by placing your feet and hands on the mat, keeping your spine and legs straight. Lift your glutes up as high as you can while maintaining a straight back. In this position, you should feel a gentle stretch in your calves.

2. Slowly place your right knee on the mat between your hands and position your right ankle between your left leg and left arm. Keep your chest up. You should feel a stretch in your right glute as you get into this position - See the second image for a clearer understanding.

3. Lastly, breathe out completely and bring your chest close to your knee, using your arms for support if needed, until the chest touches the inside of your knee. Hold this position for a full breath.

4. Come back to the initial position and repeat on the other side. Repeat for the mentioned reps alternating sides.

Note:

If the position shown in Step 3 (last photo) seems too hard, just aim to bring your chest close to the floor. If you can't do it right away, that's okay. With practice, you'll improve your hip flexibility and make your movements smoother by releasing unnecessary tension.

Focus on each step and every small movement of your body as you do this exercise - there's no need to rush through it.

If you have any issues downloading the QR code or if it does not open, please email me at somatictrainingplan@gmail.com, and I will assist you.

SIDE CHEST STRETCH

This exercise helps enhance flexibility in the chest and shoulders. Remember to breathe deeply to release tension. It also aids in improving your posture and aligning your body properly.

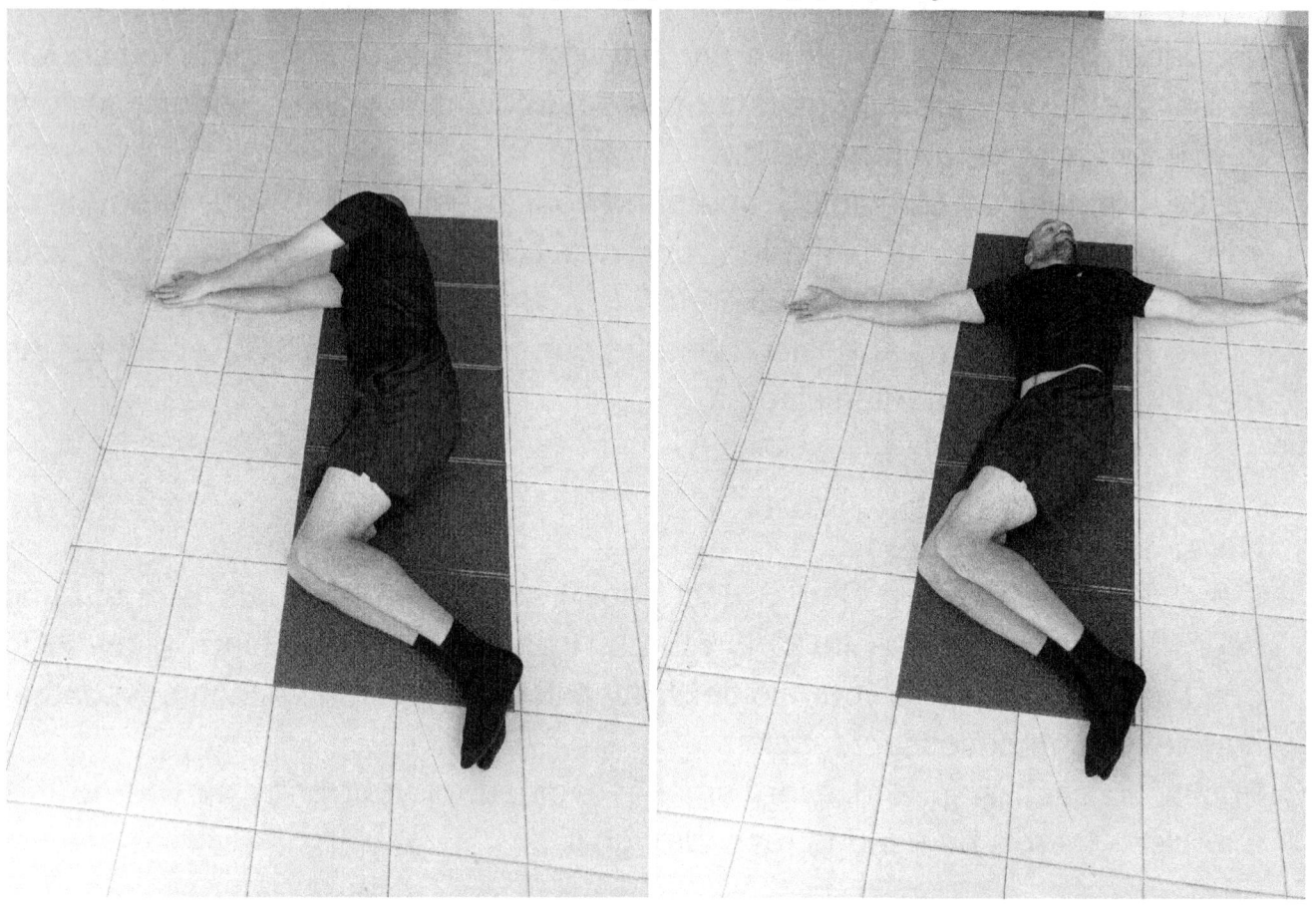

Step 1 - *Starting position*   **Step 2** - *Imagine drawing a semicircle in the air with your left hand.*

If you have any questions or doubts, feel free to contact me at

somatictrainingplan@gmail.com and I'll be happy to assist you the best I can

about somatic exercises and workouts!

How to Do it:

1. Start by lying on your right side on the floor in a fetal position. Extend your arms out in front of you on the floor.
2. Next, imagine that you are using your left hand to draw a semicircle in the air. Keep your right hand on the ground, and as you move your left hand, open up your chest.
3. Place your left hand on the floor on the other side of your body. This movement will 'open up' your chest. Hold this position for one full breath cycle, which includes both an inhale and an exhale.
4. Then, return to the starting position and repeat the movement for the specified number of repetitions.
5. Finally, switch sides by lying on your left side and repeat the same movements for the mentioned reps.

Note:

At first, you may find it difficult to fully extend your arm on the floor while opening up your chest. Don't worry; this is quite normal. Make sure to exhale deeply as you move into that position and relax your chest and shoulder area. By the second week, you should start to notice improvements!

OPENING GLUTE BRIDGE

This exercise helps strengthen your glutes and release tension in your groin area.

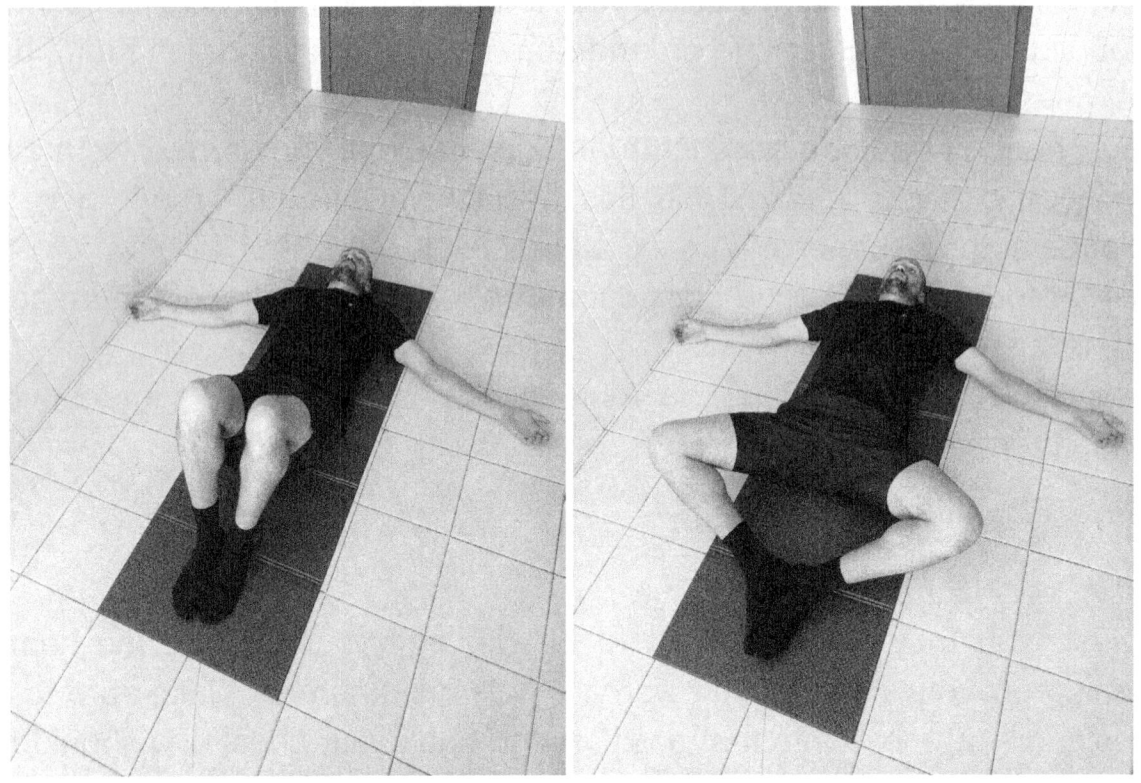

Step 1 - *Starting position*   **Step 2** - *Open up your knees.*

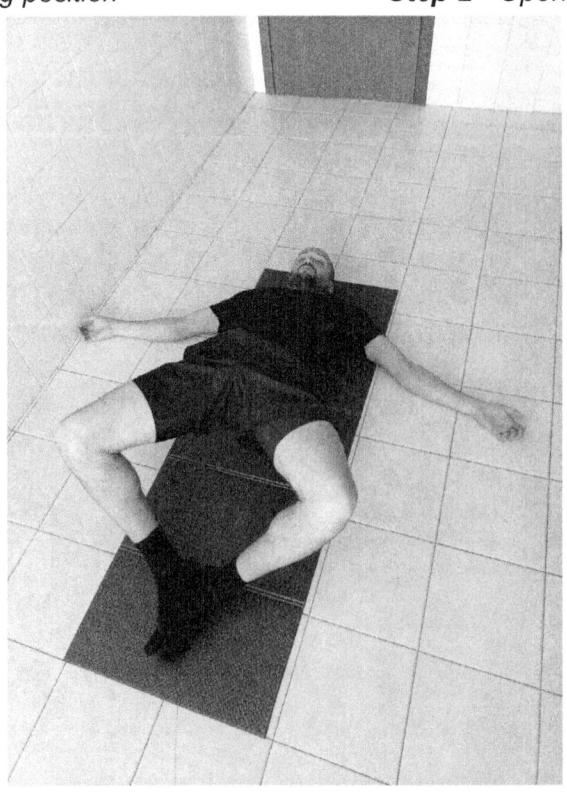

Step 3 - *Lift your hips and exhale fully.*

How to Do it:

1. Lie on your back with your knees bent and feet flat on the ground, close together. Stretch your arms out to the sides so they form a 90-degree angle with your body.
2. Breathe out gently and allow your knees to drop to the side, bringing the soles of your feet together, as shown in the second image. You'll feel a stretch in your groin. Your lower back might naturally arch a bit as you perform this step. Hold this position for 2 seconds while breathing softly.
3. Then, raise your hips while keeping your feet together, knees apart, and arms in the same position. Breath gently through your nose during the execution.
4. Lastly, slowly lower your buttocks back to the mat, bringing your knees to their starting position.
5. Your first repetition is complete. Repeat for the mentioned reps.

Note:

It is suggested to perform this exercise slowly. To maximize the benefits of the exercise, it is recommended to squeeze your glutes when pushing your hips up and hold the position.

STATIC SKIER

This exercise enhances body awareness, strength, and cardiovascular fitness while reducing stress by lowering cortisol levels.

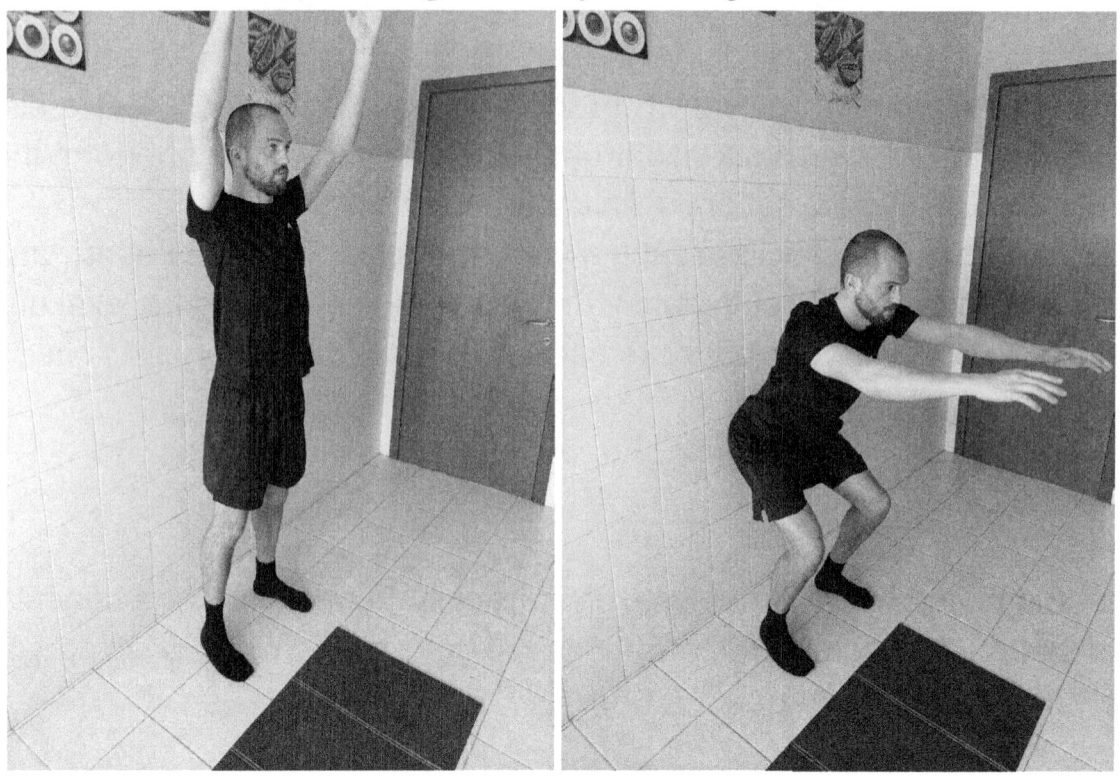

Step 1 - *Starting position with arms over head.*   **Step 2** - *Squat down and extend arms forward.*

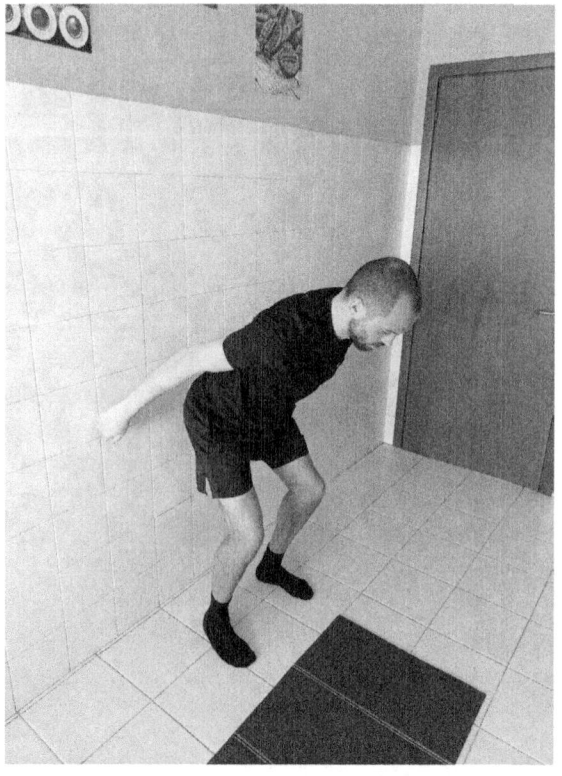

Step 3 - *Swing your hands backward releasing all the tension accumulated.*

How to Do it:

1. Stand with your feet slightly wider than shoulder-width apart, and stretch your arms above your head.
2. Lower your hands down and bend your knees, pushing your buttocks back.
3. Swing your hands backward and bend your knees until they're close to a 90-degree angle, bringing your chest close to your thighs as if you were skiing - exhale fully as you do so.
4. Go back to the starting position and repeat the movement for the mentioned seconds. Breathe in through your nose before starting again.

Note:

The key focus here is to imagine that all your tension and anxiety are in your hands. As you do the movement, push that tension away from you. Exhale while you move, then inhale when you return to the starting position.

The faster you do it, the harder it gets. While there are three steps shown, the aim is to do them so smoothly that the exercise doesn't seem like it is made by different steps.

In the 28-day plan, alternating between gentle and intense exercises helps flush toxins from your body and release negative thoughts and emotional stress.

SIDE LUNGE RELAXATION

This exercise is excellent for improving both flexibility and strength. As you stretch to one side, focusing on your breathing can help release tension.

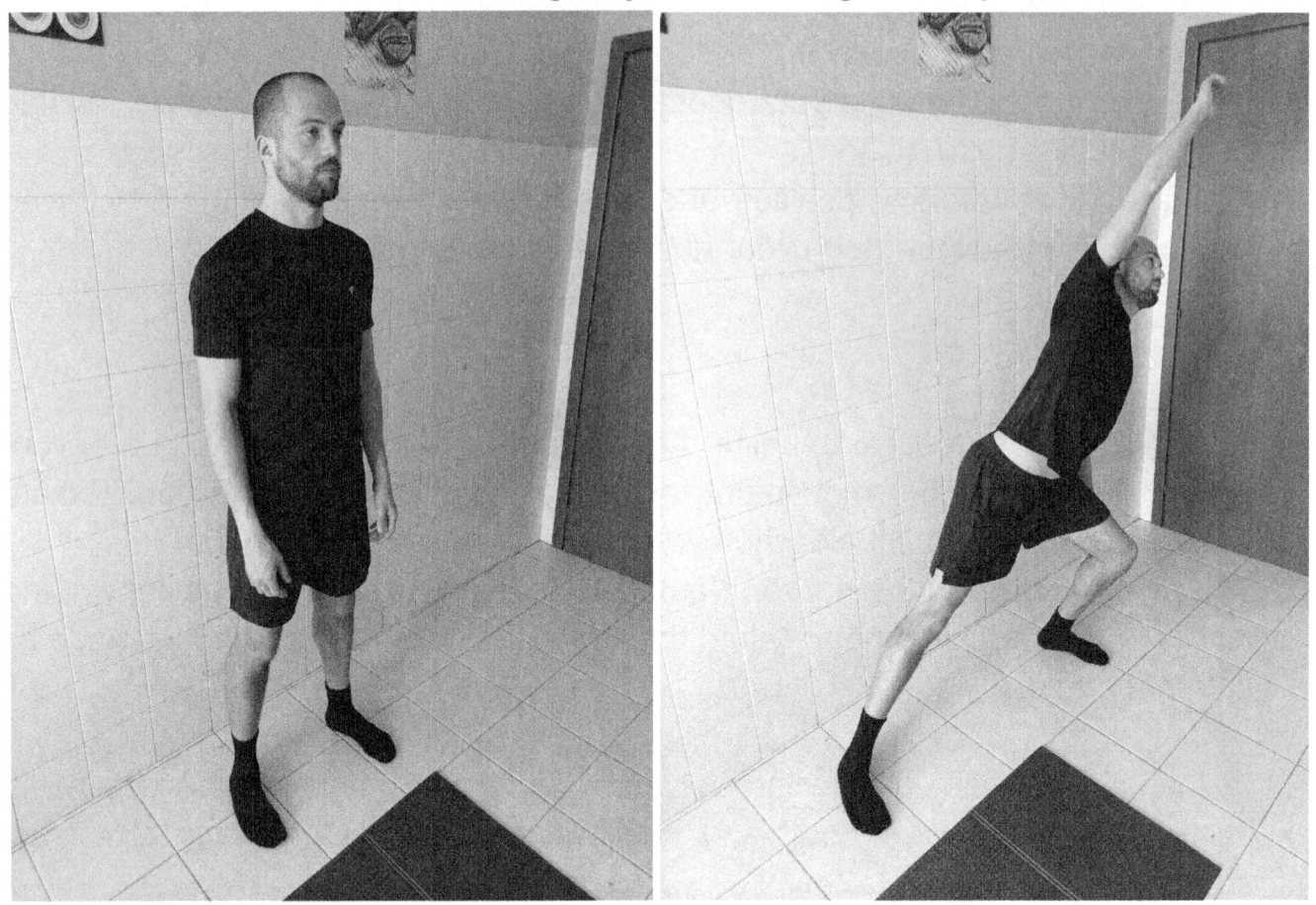

Step 1 - *Starting position.*   **Step 2** - *Lunge on one side and extend your arm as shown.*

How to Do it:

1. Stand with your arms close to your body. Take a gentle breath out before you start moving.
2. Take a step to the left with your left foot, bending your left knee while keeping your right leg straight.
3. Then, reach with your right hand over your left side, aiming to go as high and wide as possible while leaning to the left. Hold this position for two seconds, exhaling as you reach the position.
4. Lastly, slowly return to the starting position and repeat on the other side
5. Perform the movement for the mentioned reps, alternating sides.

Note:

Control your breathing, take the exercise slowly, and focus on your muscles and how you feel. You might feel a burning sensation in your left thigh and glute, as well as a stretch on the right side of your back. That's a normal sensation during this exercise. Do not force the exhale - it does not have to be long or necessarily more powerful than a normal exhale through the mouth This is worth mentioning, as many people might think otherwise.

WAVING SPINE

Exercises that move your spine help you become more flexible, lessen pain, and strengthen the connection between your mind and body.

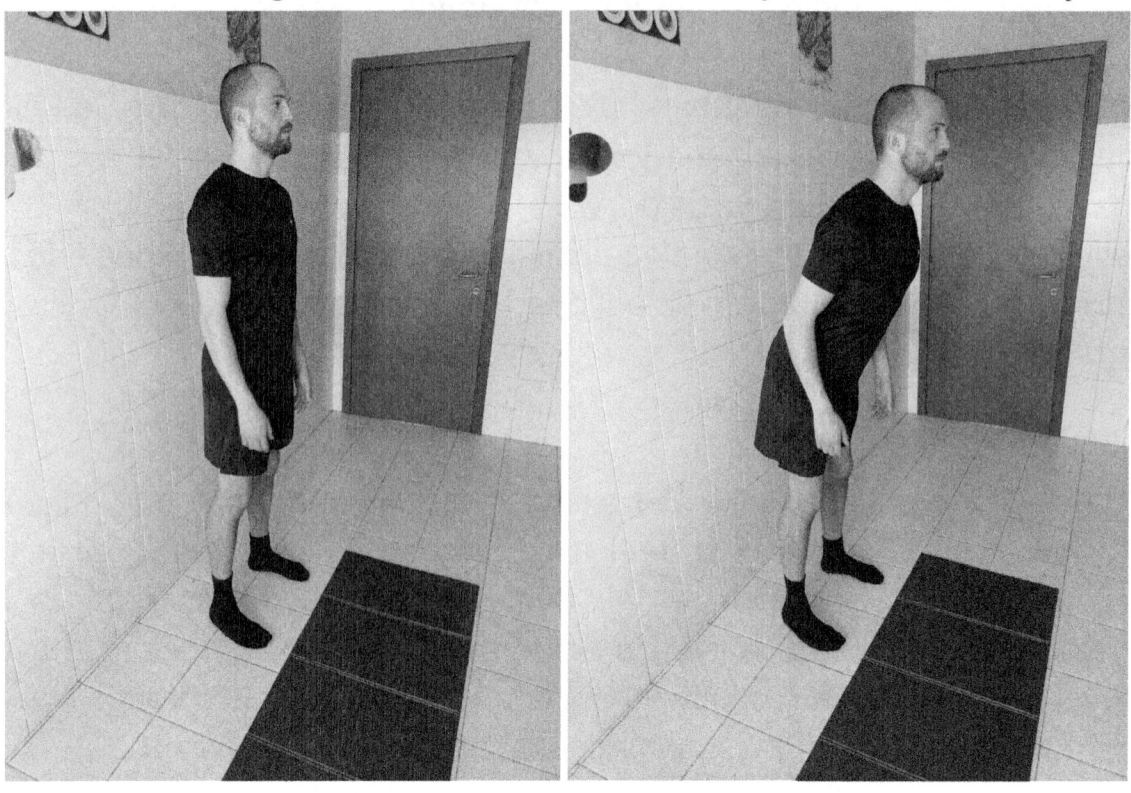

Step 1- *Starting position.*

Step 2 - *Wave your head and chest forward.*

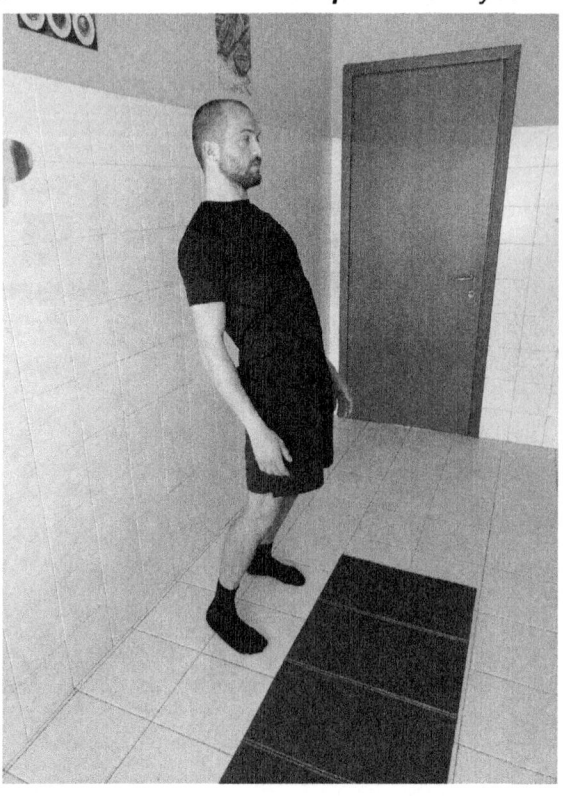

Step 3 - *Move smoothly your belly forward, continuing this waving motion.*

How to Do it:

1. Start by standing up straight with your arms at your sides and your whole body forming a straight line.
2. Next, slowly and smoothly bend your chest and head forward by flexing your spine.
3. Then, go back to the starting position by arching your lower back and pushing your belly forward.
4. Continue this sequence for the mentioned seconds.

Note:

Keep your posture straight and gently move your belly and then your chest forward, like a wave, while flexing your spine. Remember, the slower and more mindful you are while doing this, the better you'll feel afterward.

LYING KNEE UP

This exercise is great for making your body more flexible and easing tension.

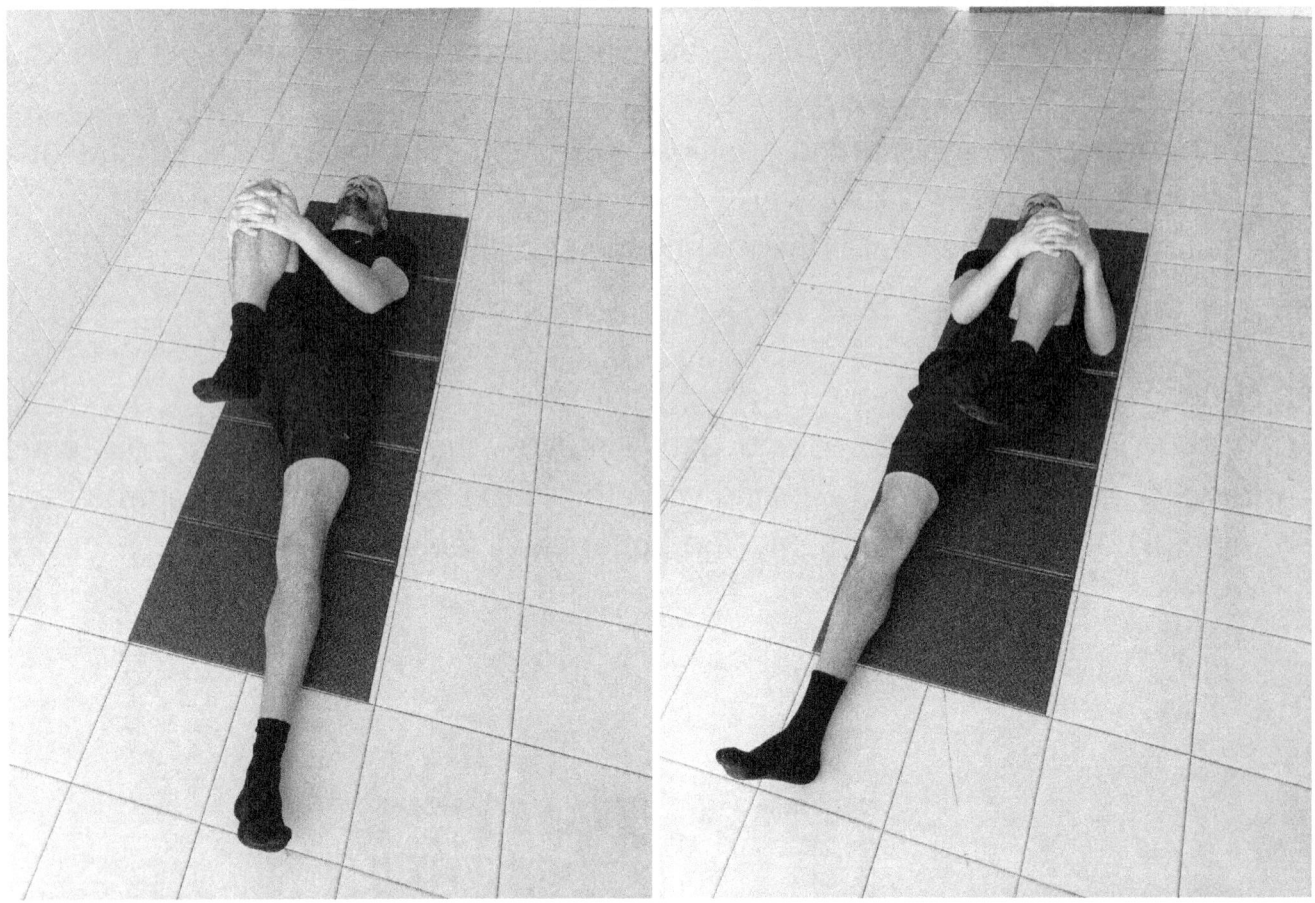

Step 1 - *Hug your right knee to your chest for 3 seconds.*   **Step 2** - *Then, repeat on the other side.*

How to Do it:

1. Lie on your back with your left leg straight on the mat and the right knee bent, hugging it close to your chest. Relax your shoulders and neck. Hold this position for 3 seconds while breathing out completely through your mouth.
2. Switch legs. Lower your right leg first, then lift your left leg up. Perform this movement slowly. Hold the position for 3 seconds while performing a full breath cycle.
3. Repeat the movement for the mentioned reps, alternating sides.

Note:

To get the best results, go slow. Remember to breathe out through your mouth. This is an awesome exercise to become more flexible. Do not worry if it's challenging to bring your knee close to your chest while keeping your back down. Just try to keep your back flat and bring your knee as close as you can while focusing on your breath and relaxing fully. You'll get better with practice.

LEG OPENED RELEASE

Complete relaxation and hip opening with this simple and gentle stretch.

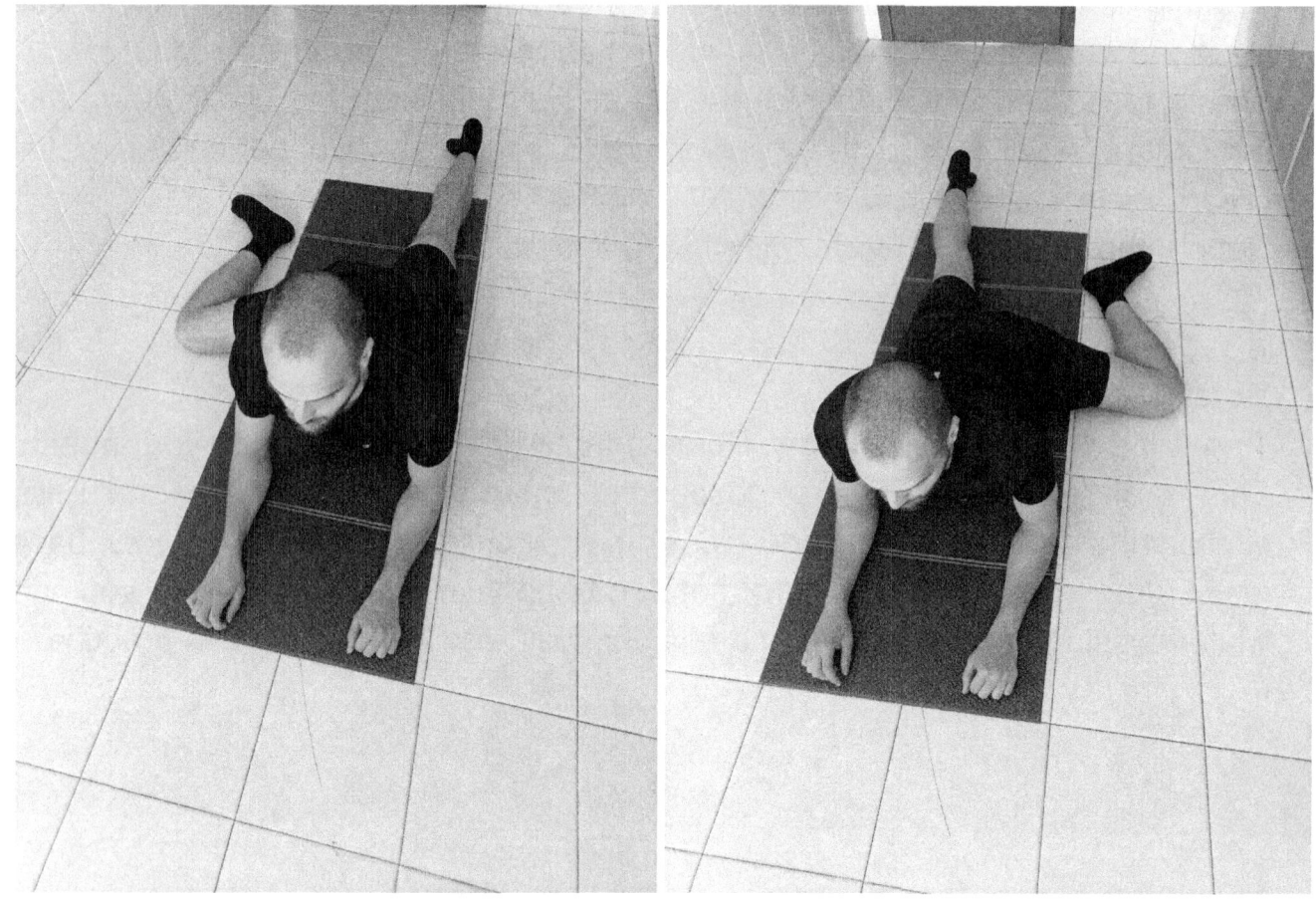

Step 1 - *Open your right hip and breathe deeply to relax.*   **Step 2** - *Perform on the other side.*

How to Do it:

1. Lie on your stomach with your right leg opened up and your right knee bent at 90°. Place your forearm on the floor and exhale deeply through your mouth.
2. Keep this position for the mentioned seconds while inhaling gently through your nose and exhaling through your mouth (each cycle should last 5-6 seconds ideally). By doing that you will release all the tensions and stress accumulated in your body.
3. Lastly, repeat on the other side.

Note:

This static exercise aims to help you release all the tension and stress accumulated in your body. Most of our stress, trauma, and tension are carried in our hips. As you assume this position, not only will your hips become more flexible, but you will also feel better from focusing on your breathing and releasing stress and tension with every exhale.

Also, do not force your breath cycle too much - some people might want to extend inhale and exhale longer hoping it will have more benefits. While that may be true for experts, it's not necessary to inhale or exhale for longer if you're not comfortable, especially in the first few weeks you're doing these exercises..

WALKING PLANK

Great core exercise to strengthen your core as well as improve the body-mind connection and coordination.

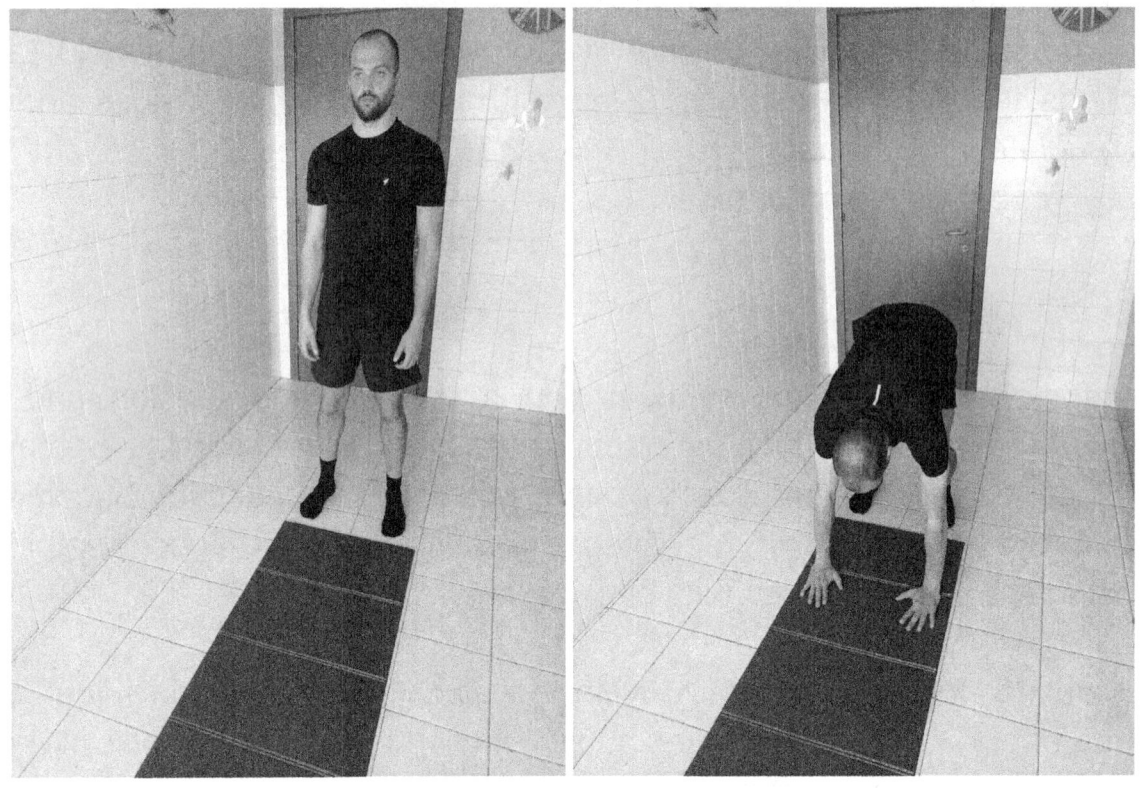

Step 1 - *Standing in front of the mat.*   **Step 2** - *Place your hands on the mat.*

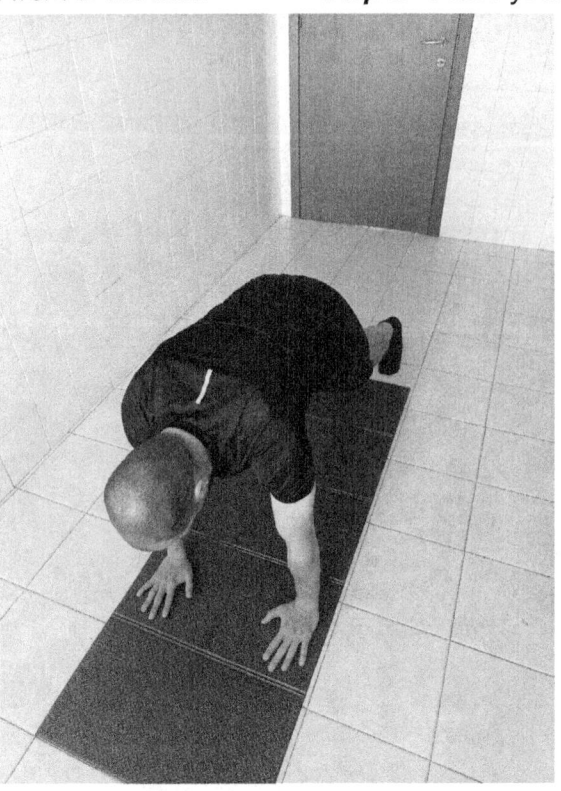

Step 3 - *Get in a plank position. Then, come back into the starting position and repeat.*

How to Do it:

1. Start in a standing position in front of your mat.
2. From there bend your back and reach the floor with your hands. Feel free to slightly bend your knees as you do so - see Step 2.
3. Then, walk your hands forward almost to get in a plank position - see Step 3.
4. Then, slowly come back until your arms are close to your body.
5. From there, stand back up and exhale fully, releasing all the stress accumulated in your body.
6. This is one rep. Repeat this sequence for the mentioned reps.

Note:

I suggest performing this movement slowly and with control to ensure you engage your core in each step of the exercise and get the most out of it, both physically and spiritually. The slower and more controlled you perform it, the more present you will necessarily be.

BODY CIRCLES

Great for opening up the hips as well as improving body control.

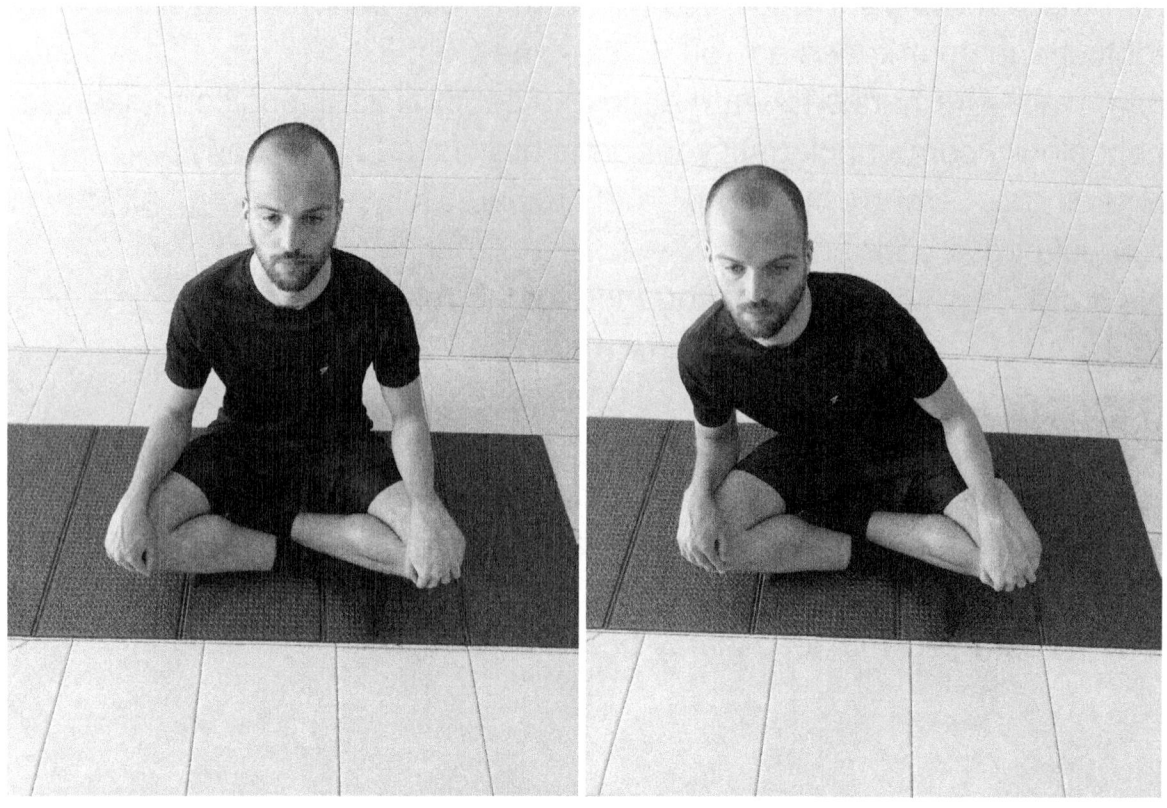

Step 1 - *Sit cross-legged with hands on your knees.*   **Step 2** - *Gently sway your hips and trunk to one side.*

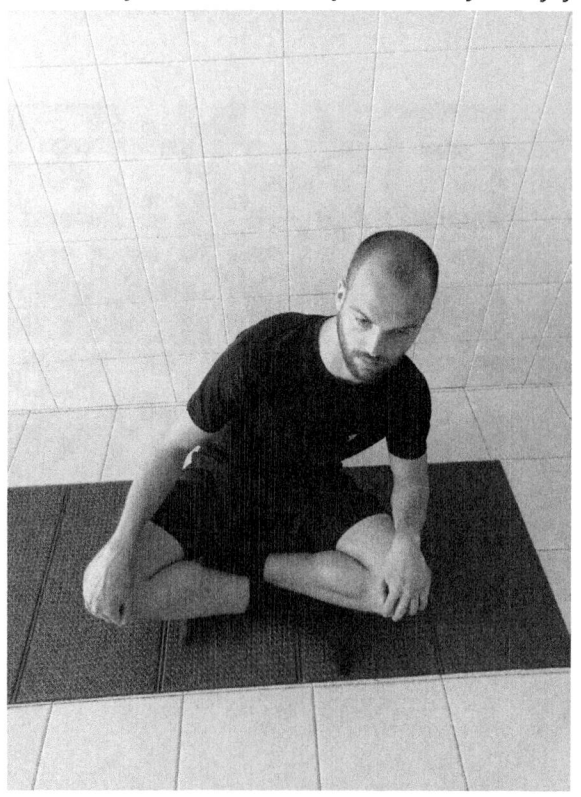

Step 3 - *Keep moving your hip in a circular way exploring new ranges of motion, whilst breathing softly.*

How to Do it:

1. Start sitting on the mat with your legs crossed and hands on your knees. Take a deep breath for relaxation.
2. Gently move your upper body in a circular motion as shown in the image (and in the video).
3. Repeat it for the mentioned reps at a slow pace. Keep breathing gently as you do so.
4. Lastly, switch directions and repeat it for the same amount of rep.

Note:

I suggest that during the practice, you be fully present with your body and emotions, and accept whatever feelings arise, knowing that through this practice, they will eventually vanish.

ROLL DOWN

A fantastic exercise to release negativity whilst improving the body-mind connection.

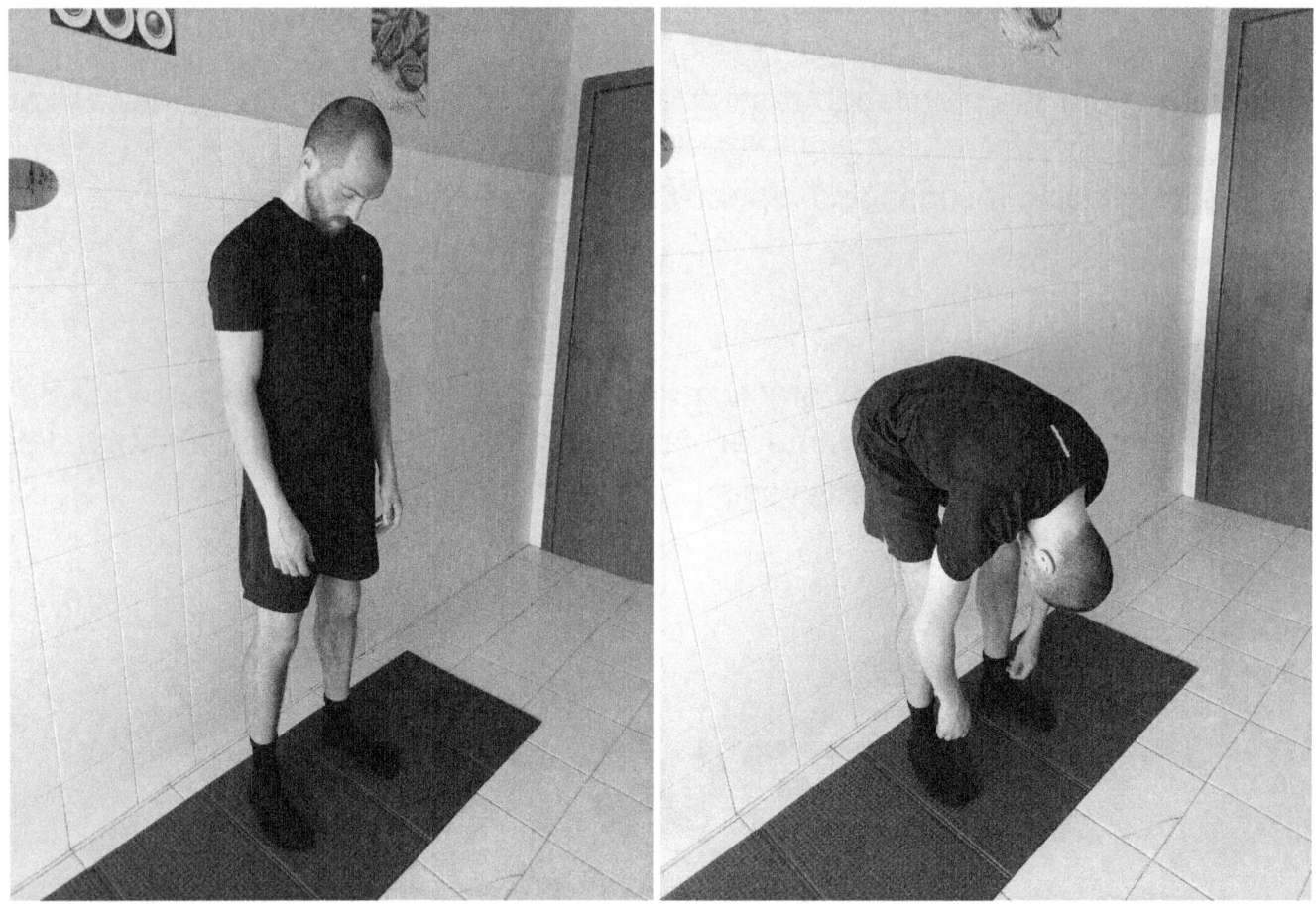

Step 1 - *Stand, tuck your chin, and roll down slowly.*   **Step 2** - *Bounce at the bottom a few times, then return to start.*

How to Do it:

1. Start by rolling down from your head, one vertebra at a time, slowly opening up the entire posterior chain of your body.

2. When you reach your legs, feel free to slightly bend your knees if you experience too much stress on the back of your legs.

3. Once you've rolled down completely, bounce a few times to gauge your body's response. Exhale fully through your mouth to release all the tension in your body.

4. Finally, slowly return to the starting position. Each repetition should take anywhere between 10 and 20 seconds.

5. Repeat for the specified number of repetitions.

Note:

I suggest visualizing your spine as it gently bends forward during the rolling. While 'bouncing,' focus on letting go of every tension, thought, or stress you are carrying. Completely relax your upper body to maximize the benefits of the exercise.

UP & DOWN

This exercise routine combines lower-body workouts with cardio exercises, which can help with weight loss. It also improves coordination.

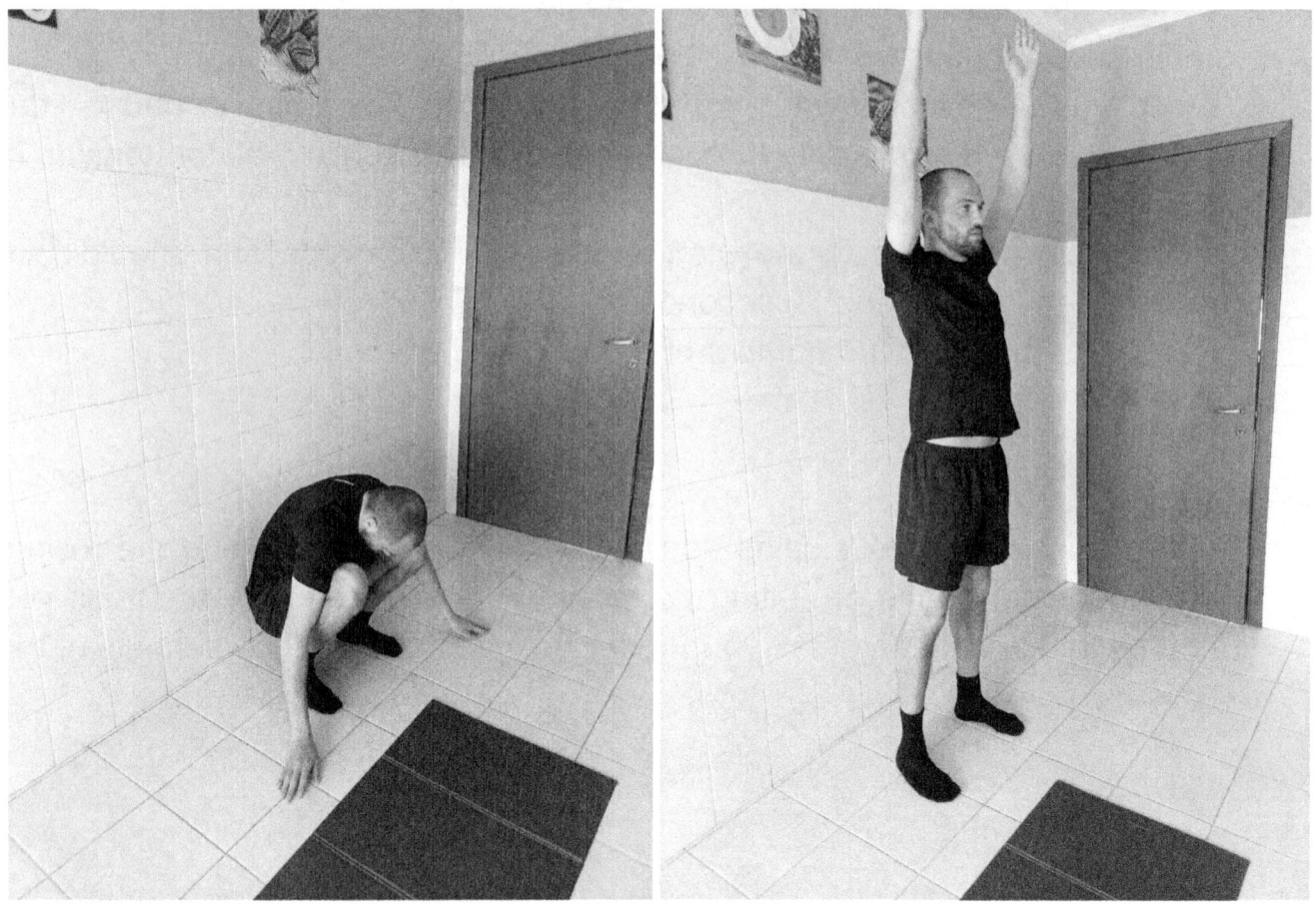

Step 1 - *Squat down with hands on the floor.*   **Step 2 -** *Stand back up, lift your arms, exhale fully.*

How to Do it:

1. Start by getting into a deep squat position with your hands on the floor and breathe in through your nose.
2. Then, stand up straight with your arms extended overhead as if you're mimicking a flower blooming. Breathe out completely, imagining you're releasing all the built-up tension.
3. Lastly, come back to the starting position and repeat for the mentioned reps.

Note:

This exercise is quite challenging for your cardiovascular system. Ideally, try to do it without stopping. You don't need to go fast; a steady and controlled movement for the specified number of repetitions works really well.

HIP BUTTERFLY SHAKE

Great exercise to shake & release trauma and tension from hips & inner thighs.

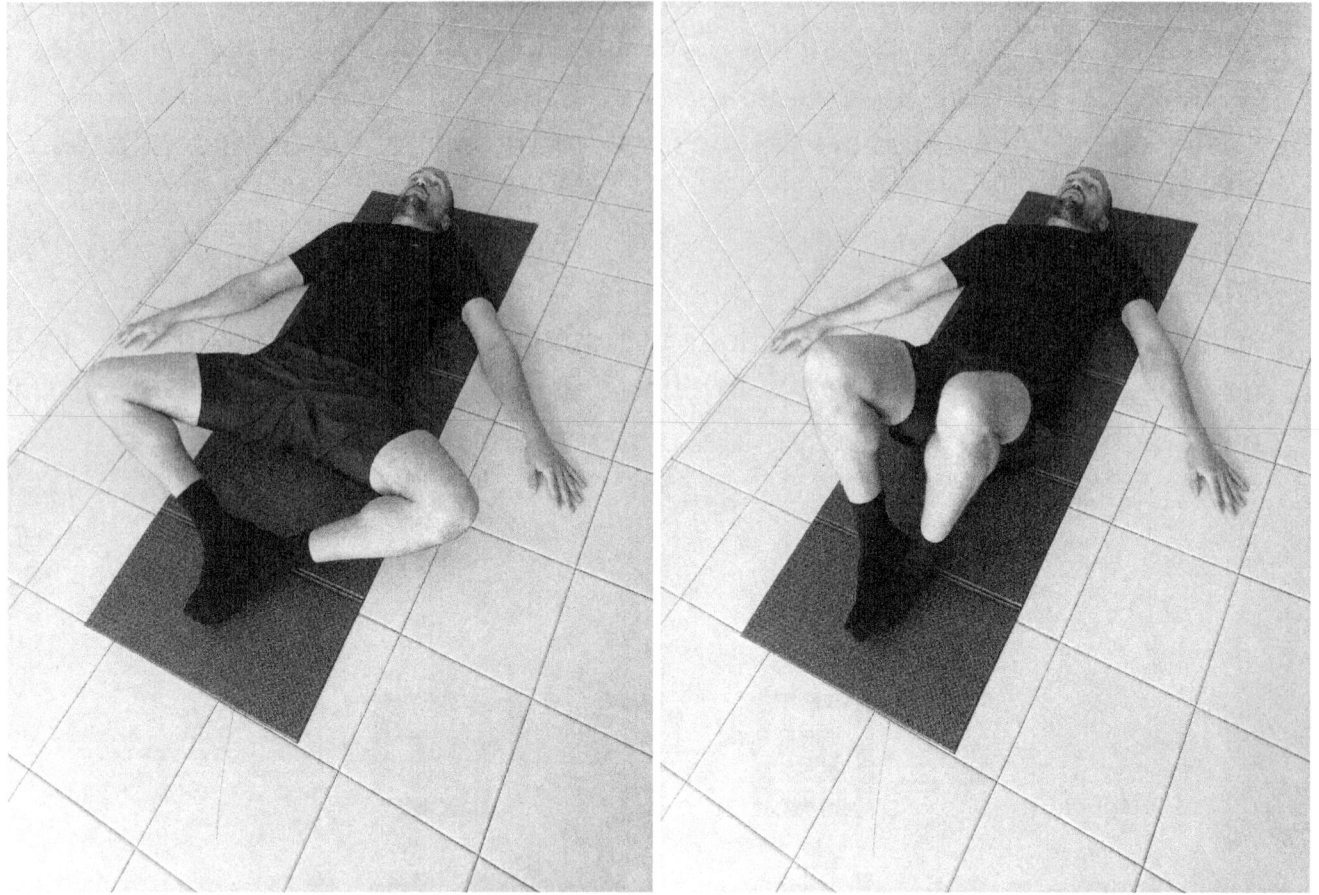

Step 1 - Lie back, arms aside, knees bent outward.   *Step 2 - Press feet together and lift knees until they touch.*

If you have any questions or doubts, feel free to contact me at somatictrainingplan@gmail.com, and I'll be happy to assist you the best I can about somatic exercises and workouts!

How to Do it:

1. Lie down on your back with your arms at your sides and the soles of your feet together. Open your knees to the sides.
2. From there, press your feet together as you slowly bring the knees towards each other (You might shake a bit while doing so). Keep breathing softly.
3. Once the knees are close to each other, return to the starting position, releasing all tension. Exhale completely through your mouth.
4. Repeat for the specified number of repetitions.

Note:

Some people might also experience goosebumps or feel heaviness in their chest... Although this is not very common, it's worth mentioning in case it happens to you. If you do experience these sensations, know that it's completely okay, especially at the beginning! However, if you have any physical concerns, it is highly recommended to consult your doctor before continuing with this training program.

SHIFTING HIPS

Here's a good exercise to help get rid of the trauma and negativity that builds up inside your body from feelings that you haven't dealt with.

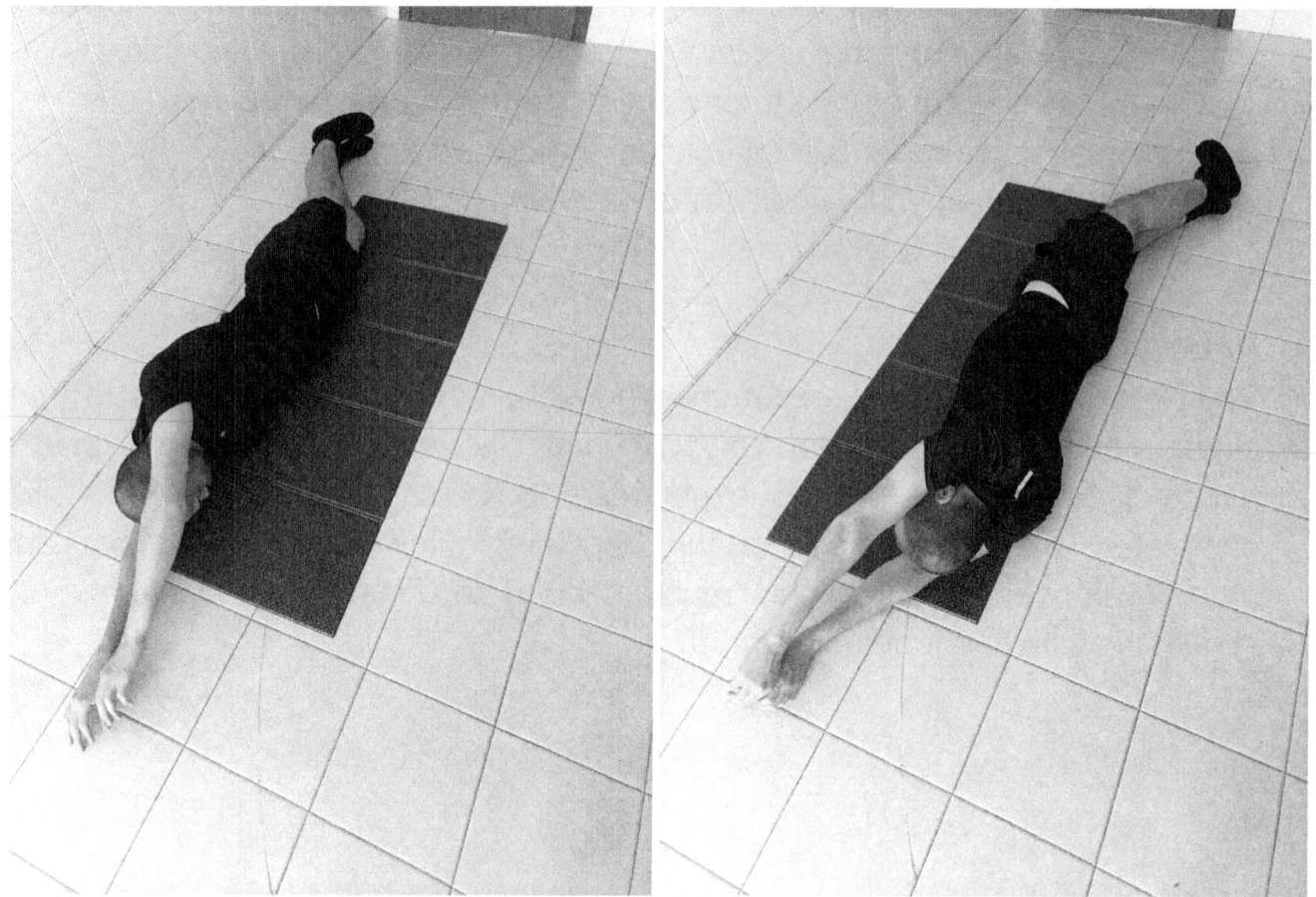

Step 1 - *Shift your body to one side.*   **Step 2** - *Then, smoothly swing to the other side.*

How to Do it:

1. Start by lying down flat on your stomach on the floor. Put your feet together and stretch your arms out in front of you.
2. Next, gently slide your hips to one side, so that your back and chest are not touching the mat. Exhale through your mouth as you do so.
3. Then, smoothly slide them to the other side.
4. Keep moving your hips from one side to the other side for the mentioned reps.

Note:

It is important to truly feel your body, especially your trunk, in contact with the floor/mat as you roll. Imagine your body as heavy and completely relaxed on the floor, gently shifting side to side and releasing all the tension built up in the body.

BENT KNEE RELAXATION

This is a great exercise for lowering high cortisol levels, which helps balance your hormones

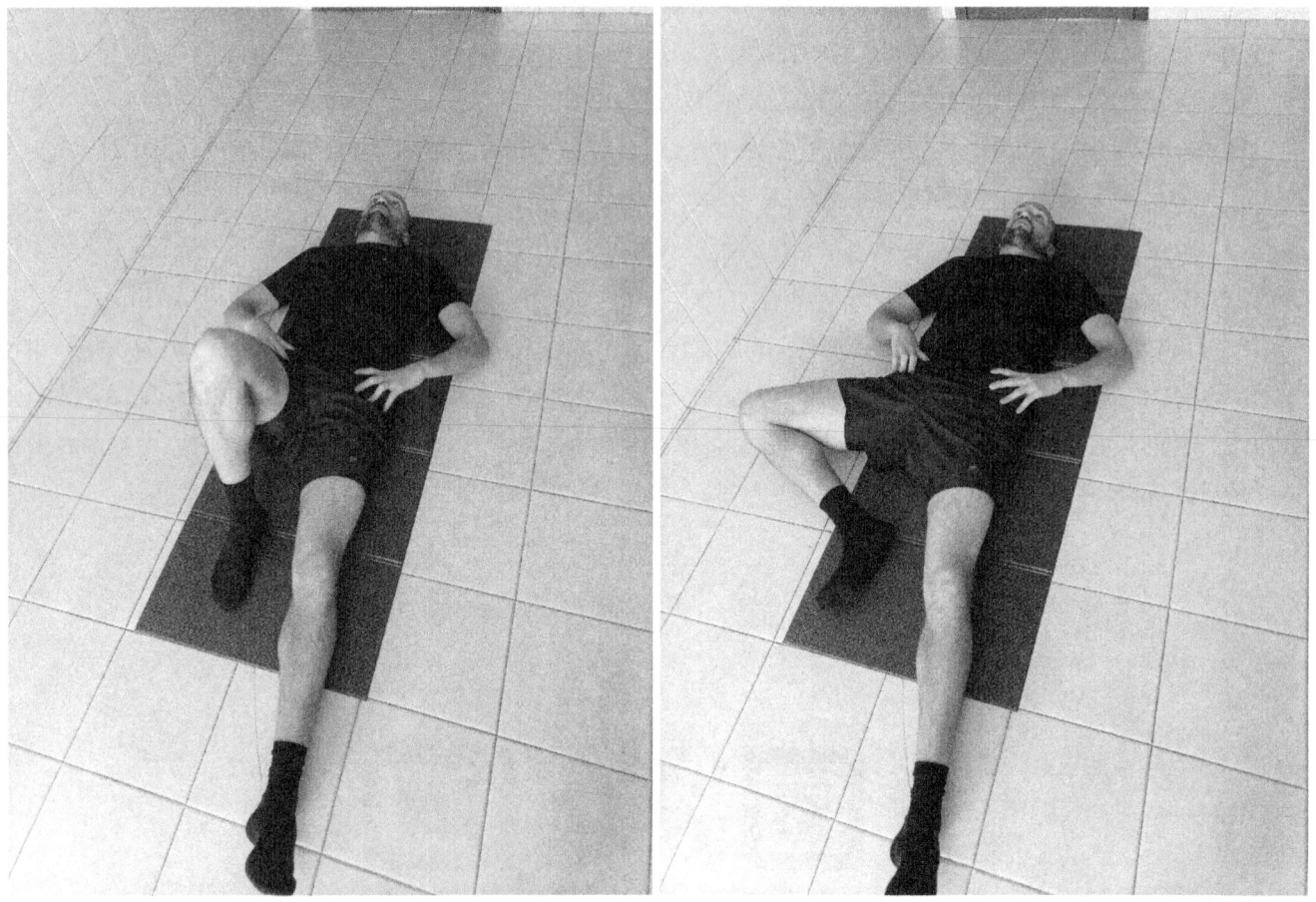

Step 1 - Lie back, arms on waist, bend right knee.　　**Step 2** - Let your knee fall out to ease hip tension.

How to Do it:

1. Lie down on your back on the mat with your hands on your waist. Keep your left leg straight and bend your right leg.
2. From there, gently lower the right leg towards the floor, as shown, while exhaling through your mouth. Hold this position for 2 seconds.
3. Then, return to the starting position while inhaling.
4. Repeat this sequence for the mentioned reps.
5. Once you finish, switch sides and repeat for the same amount of reps.

Note:

As you exhale and open up your leg, concentrate on relaxing the muscles around your hips. This will help make the exercise more effective.

OPEN & DOWN

This exercise is excellent for reducing stress and getting better balance. It's a great way to tune in and connect with your body.

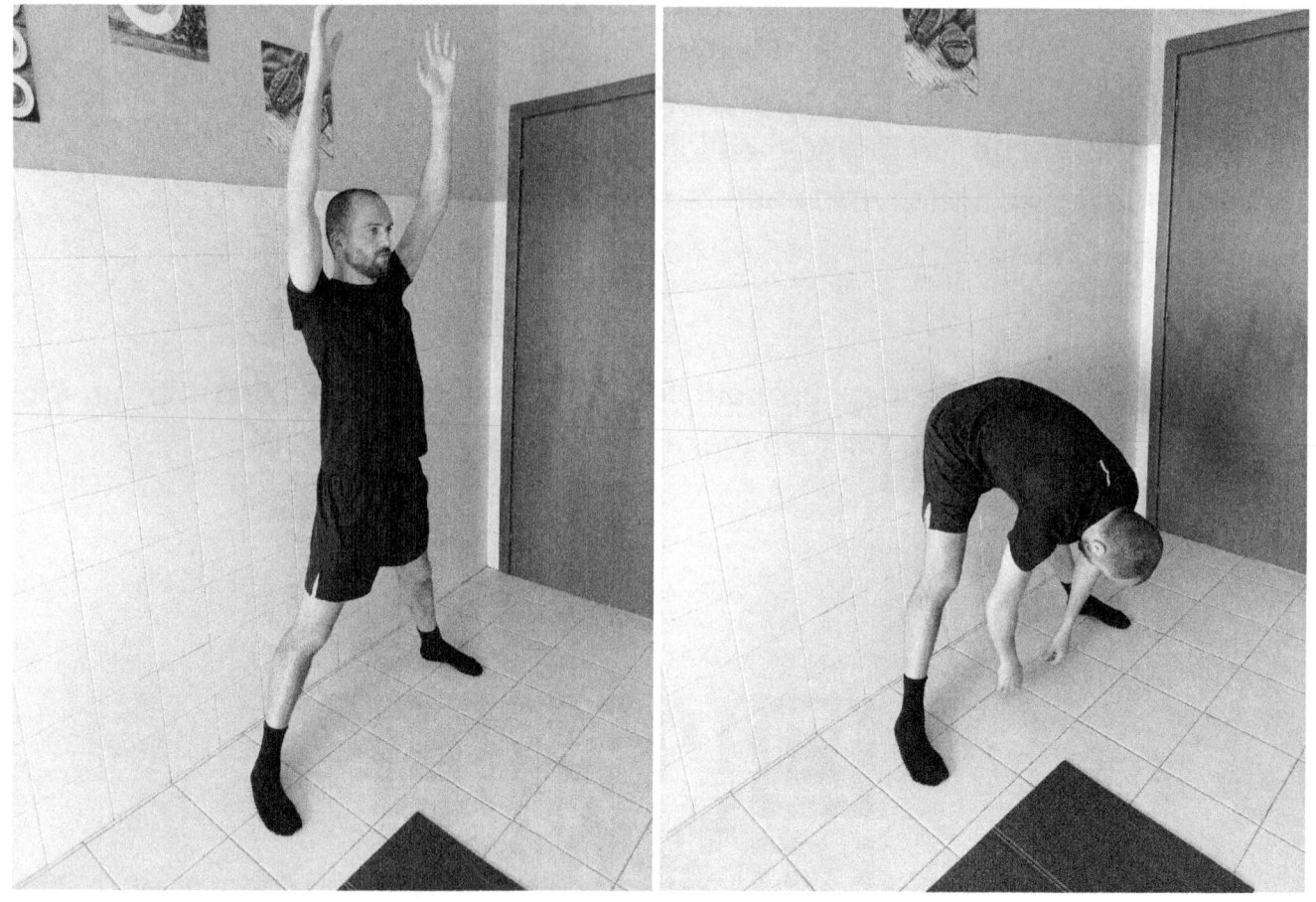

Step 1 - *Stand wide, inhale, and lift arms and chest.* **Step 2**- *Exhale, bend your back, and relax all muscles.*

How to Do it:

1. Stand with your legs apart and your arms on the sides.
2. Raise your arms over your head as you breathe in through your nose, filling your chest completely. Visualize yourself absorbing all the positive energy around you. This should only take one to two seconds.
3. Next, lower your upper body and arms towards the floor as you let go of all your emotions and muscle tension. This should take two to three seconds - Breathe out completely as you do so.
4. Then, return to the starting position and perform for the mentioned reps.

Note:

This exercise is wonderful for reconnecting with your body and finding relief with just a few deep breaths. It's best to spread your legs wider, especially when exhaling and relaxing your back.

DOWNWARD DOG

This exercise is excellent for enhancing flexibility and achieving harmony throughout your entire body.

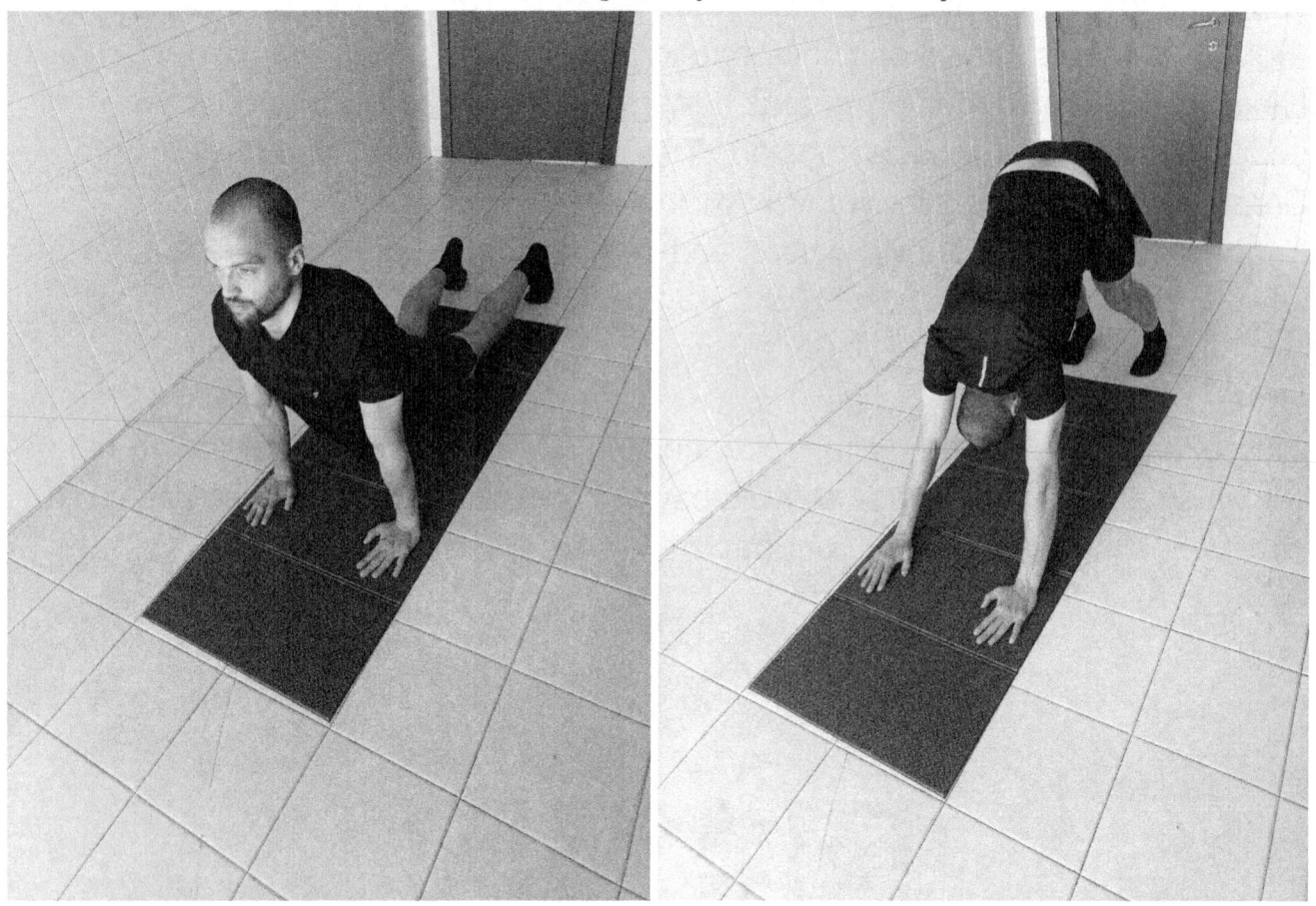

Step 1 - *Body off the floor, hands/feet on the mat, chest up.* **Step 2** - *Lift your hips and exhale fully.*

How to Do it:

1. Start on the mat with your feet and hands on the ground. Keep your body raised - Arms straight and your chest lifted (legs are not touching the floor). Breathe in while holding this position.

2. As you exhale, lift your buttocks as high as you can while keeping your feet and hands on the mat. Make sure your legs and back are straight, aiming to form a triangle shape with the mat on the other side. Hold this position for one second - Exhale fully.

3. Come back to the initial position and repeat for the mentioned reps.

Note:

Focus on your breathing and only stretch and relax the muscles that are needed. Try not to tense up your body. This exercise is great for stretching your posterior chain, which often gets tight from sitting a lot.

If you feel too much stretch in the back of your legs when you lift your hips in Step 2, you can slightly bend your knees. Eventually, you'll be able to do the exercise without bending them.

28-DAY PLAN

If you have any questions or doubts, feel free to contact me at
somatictrainingplan@gmail.com, and I'll be happy to assist you the best I
can about somatic exercises and workouts!

Day 1 - Repeat it twice.

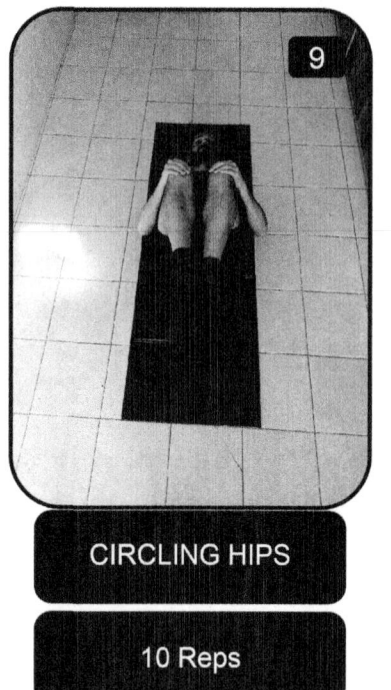

CIRCLING HIPS

10 Reps

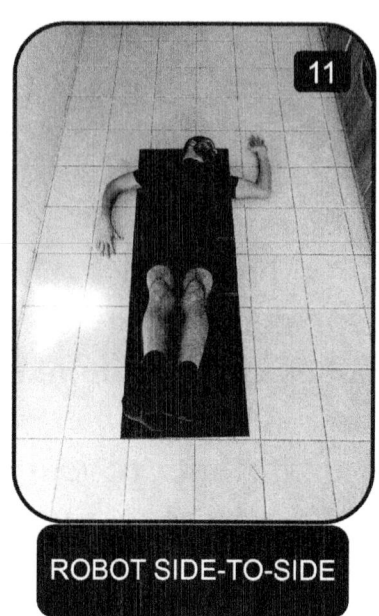

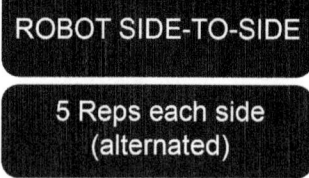

ROBOT SIDE-TO-SIDE

5 Reps each side
(alternated)

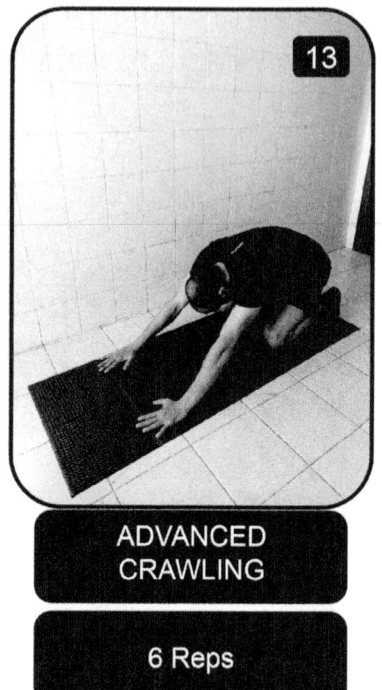

**ADVANCED
CRAWLING**

6 Reps

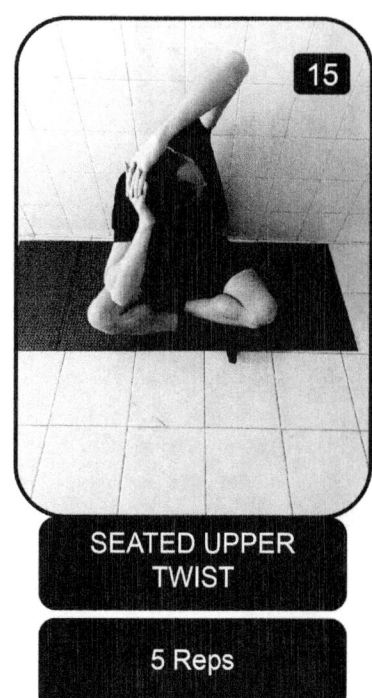

**SEATED UPPER
TWIST**

5 Reps

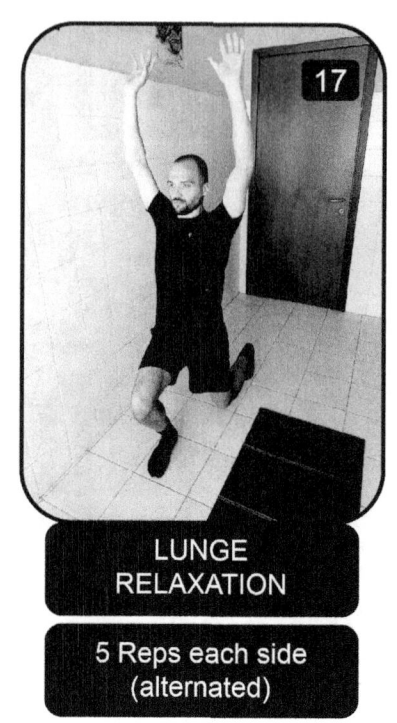

**LUNGE
RELAXATION**

5 Reps each side
(alternated)

Day 2 - Repeat it twice.

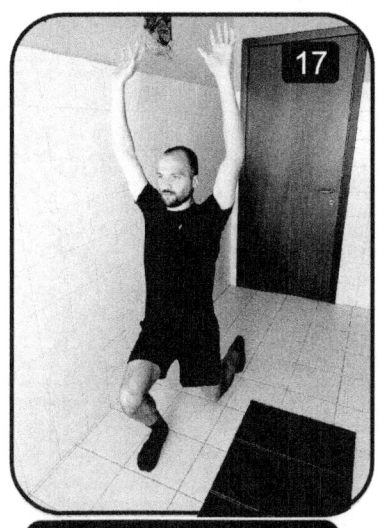

LUNGE RELAXATION

5 Reps each side (alternated)

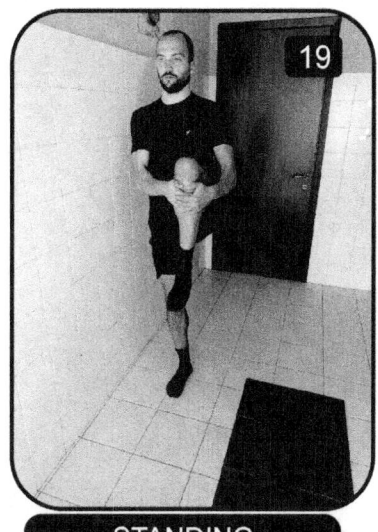

STANDING KNEE UP

5 Reps each side (alternated)

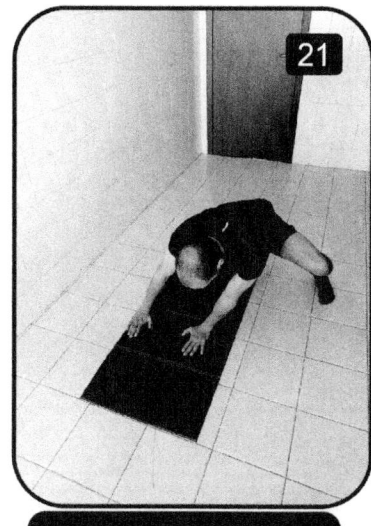

ADVANCED BODY CIRCLES

6 Reps each side

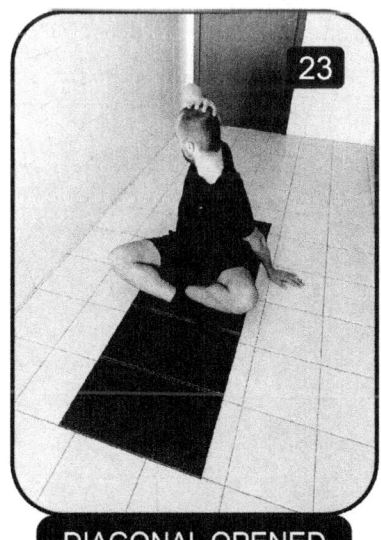

DIAGONAL OPENED TWIST

6 Reps each side

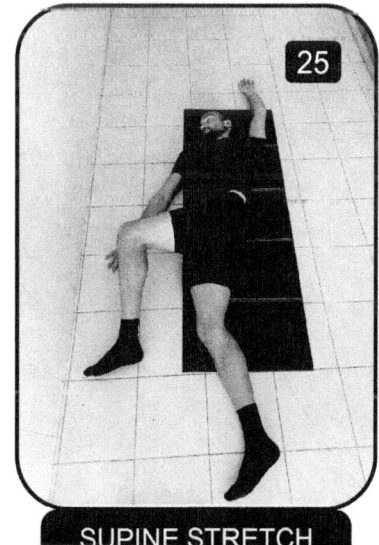

SUPINE STRETCH AND TWIST

3 Reps each side (alternated)

Day 3 - Repeat it twice.

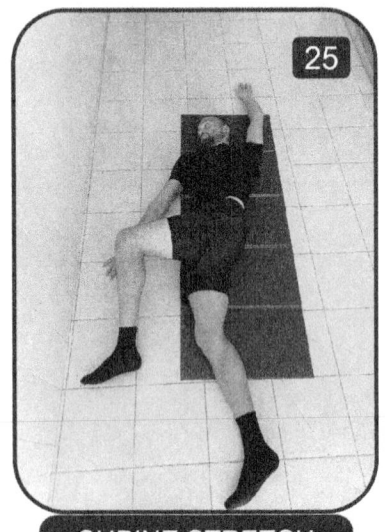

SUPINE STRETCH AND TWIST

3 Reps each side (alternated)

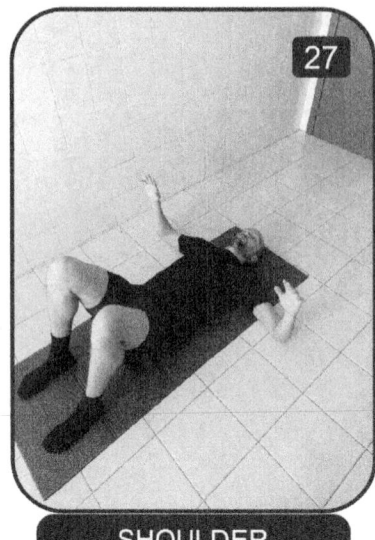

SHOULDER OPENING

6 Reps

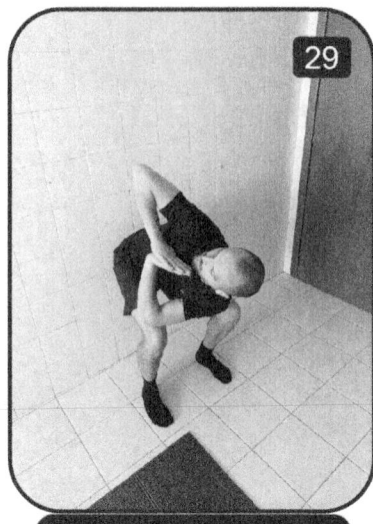

SEATED CHAIR TWIST

5 Reps each side (alternated)

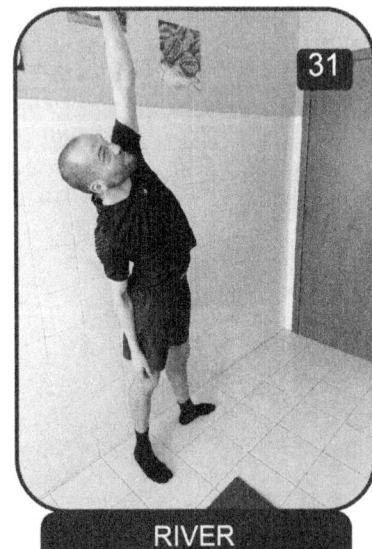

RIVER STRETCH

3 Reps each side (alternated)

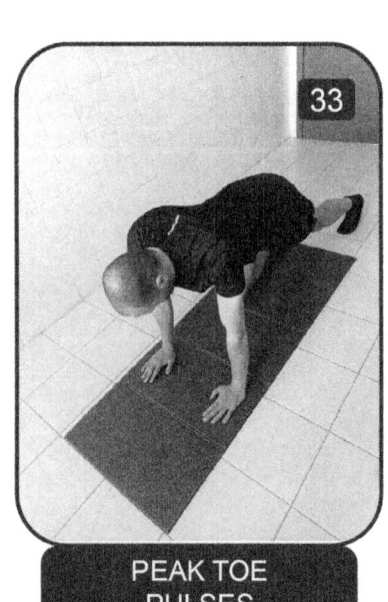

PEAK TOE PULSES

30 Seconds each side

Day 4 - Repeat it twice.

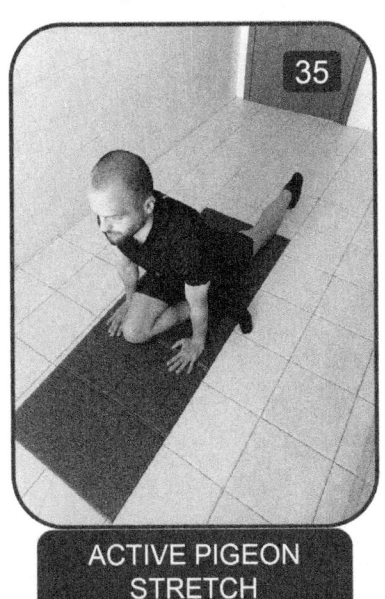

ACTIVE PIGEON STRETCH

4 Reps each side (alternated)

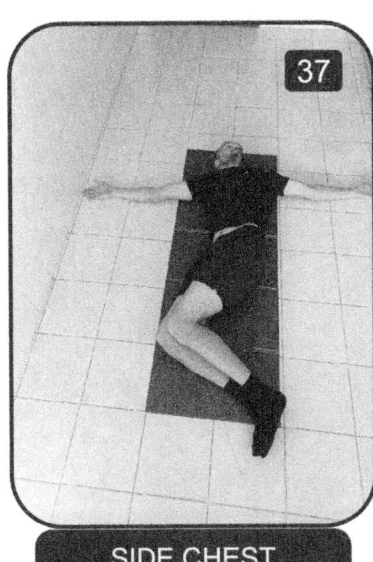

SIDE CHEST STRETCH

4 Reps each side (alternated)

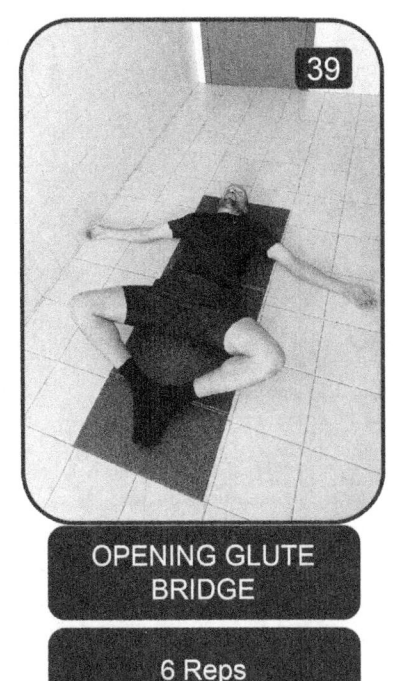

OPENING GLUTE BRIDGE

6 Reps

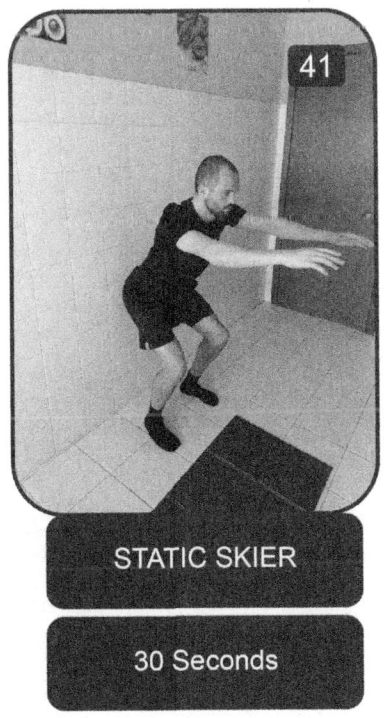

STATIC SKIER

30 Seconds

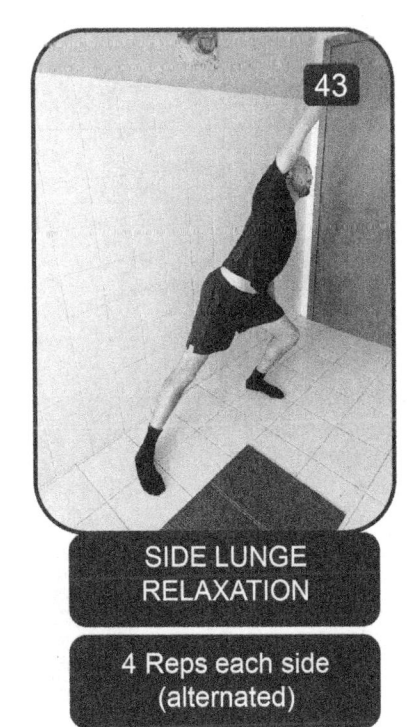

SIDE LUNGE RELAXATION

4 Reps each side (alternated)

Day 5 - Repeat it three times.

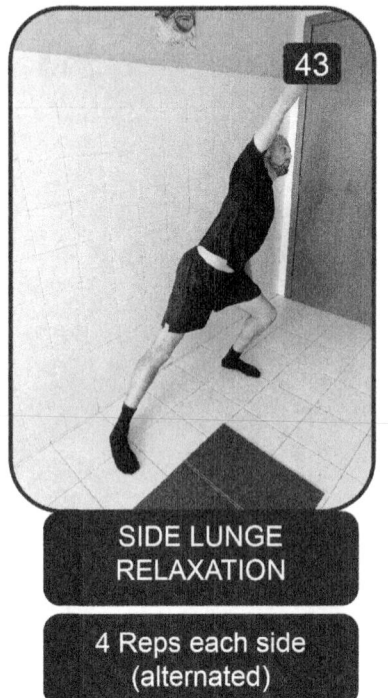

SIDE LUNGE RELAXATION

4 Reps each side (alternated)

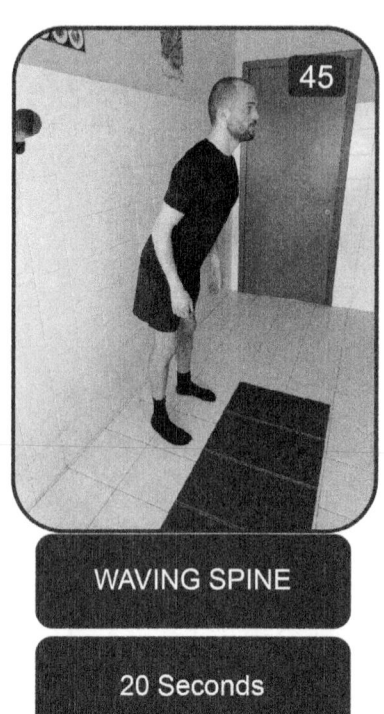

WAVING SPINE

20 Seconds

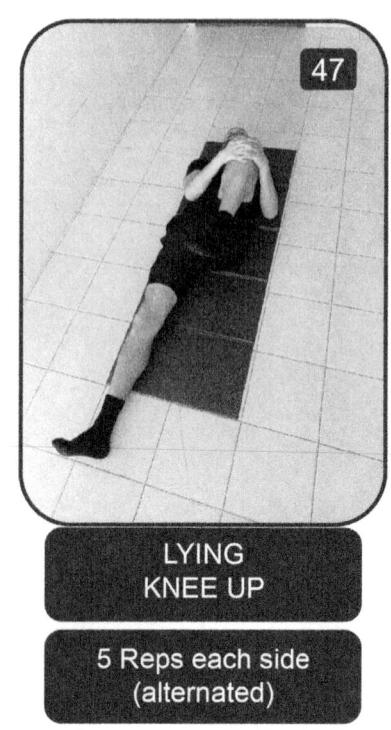

LYING KNEE UP

5 Reps each side (alternated)

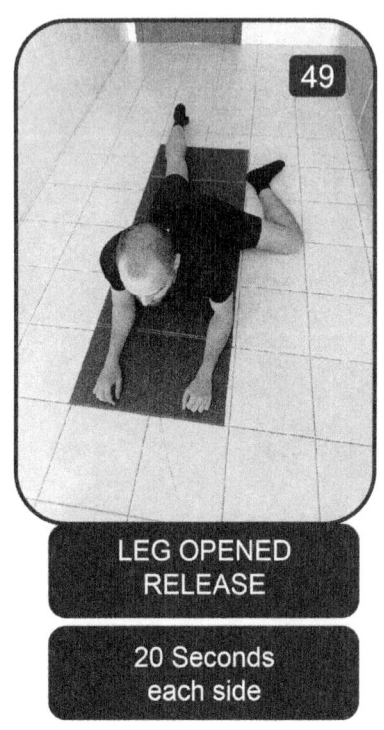

LEG OPENED RELEASE

20 Seconds each side

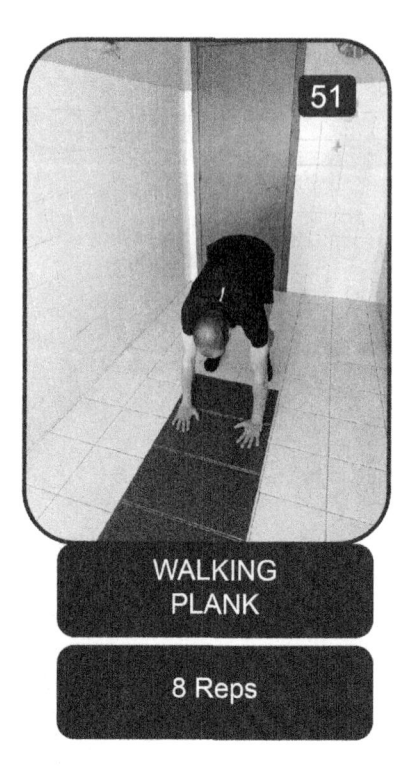

WALKING PLANK

8 Reps

Day 6 - Repeat it three times.

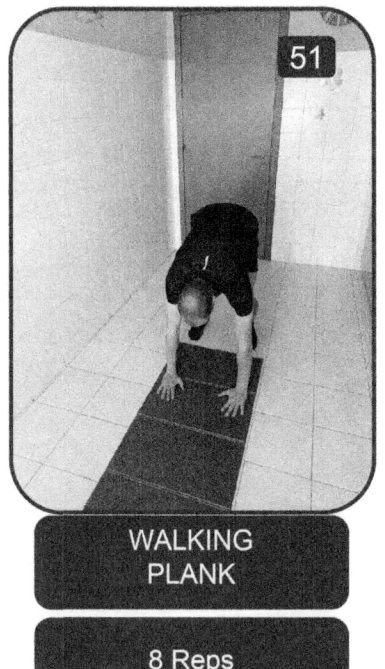

WALKING PLANK

8 Reps

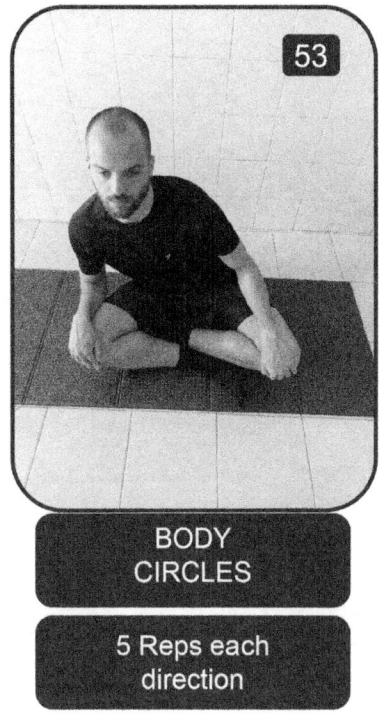

BODY CIRCLES

5 Reps each direction

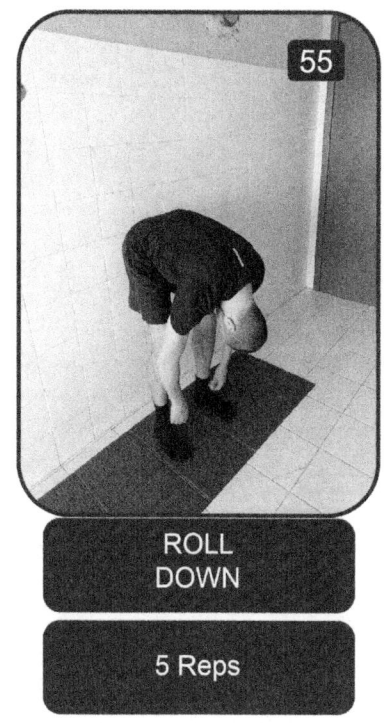

ROLL DOWN

5 Reps

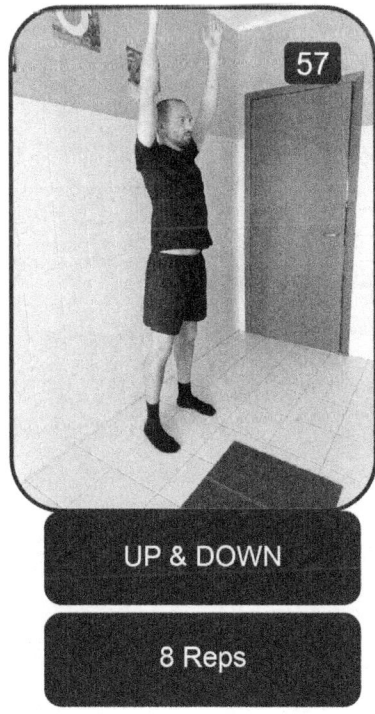

UP & DOWN

8 Reps

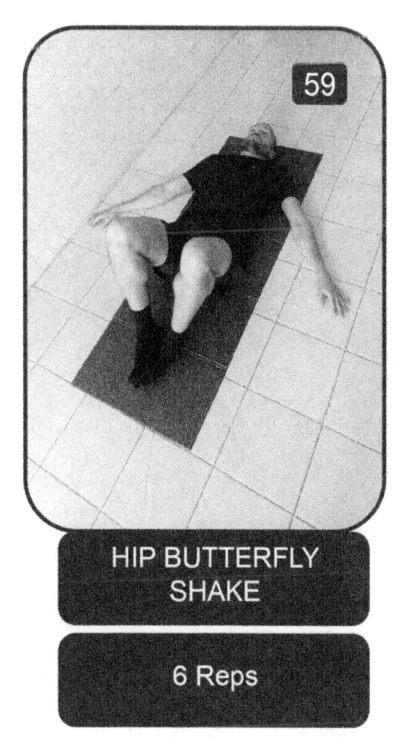

HIP BUTTERFLY SHAKE

6 Reps

Day 7 - Repeat it three times.

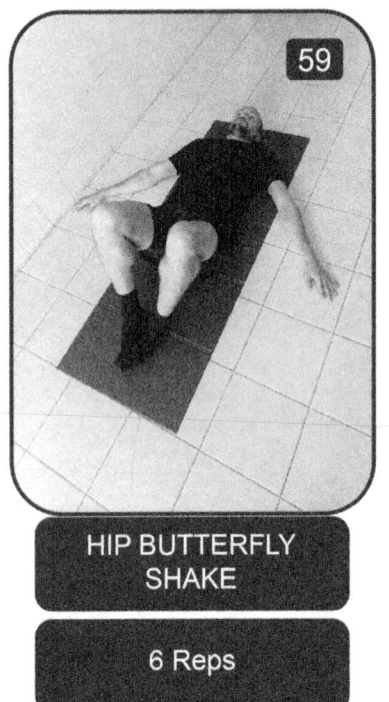

HIP BUTTERFLY SHAKE

6 Reps

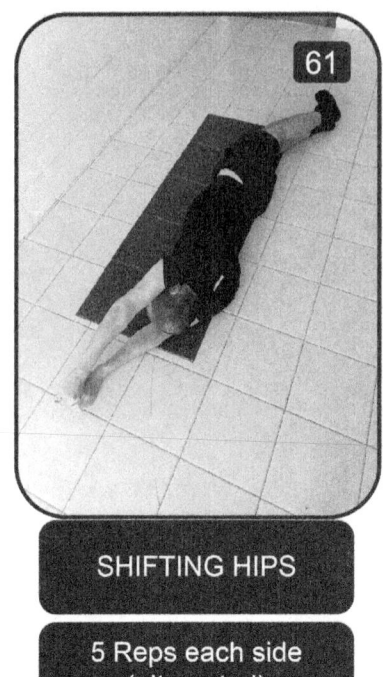

SHIFTING HIPS

5 Reps each side (alternated)

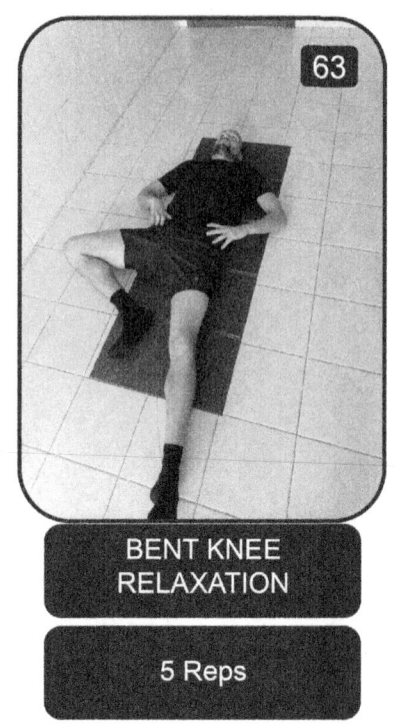

BENT KNEE RELAXATION

5 Reps

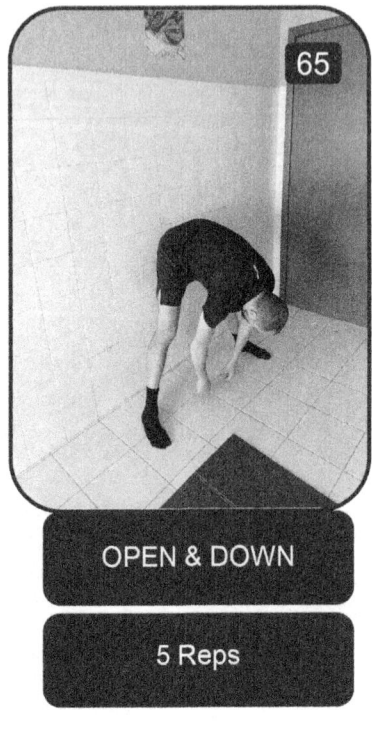

OPEN & DOWN

5 Reps

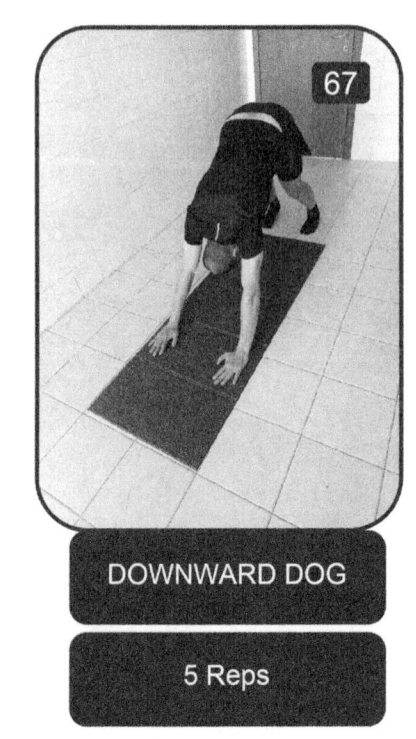

DOWNWARD DOG

5 Reps

Day 8 - Repeat it three times.

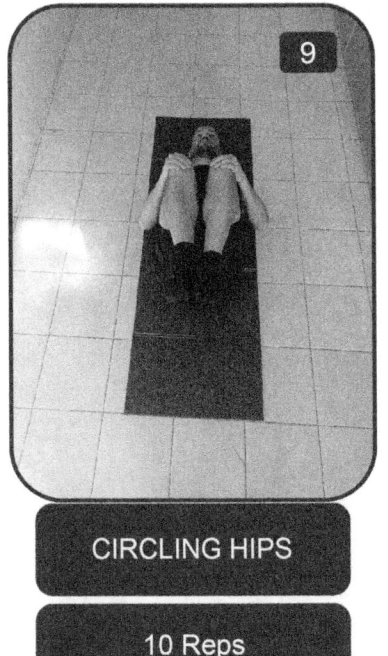

CIRCLING HIPS

10 Reps

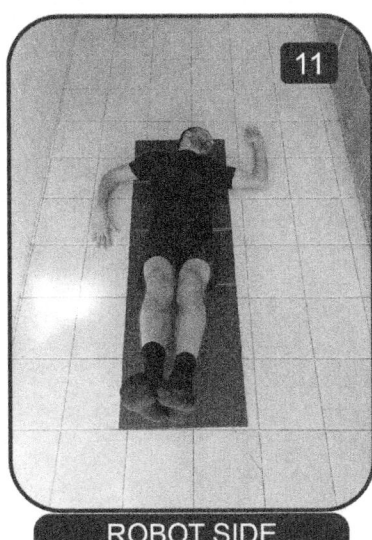
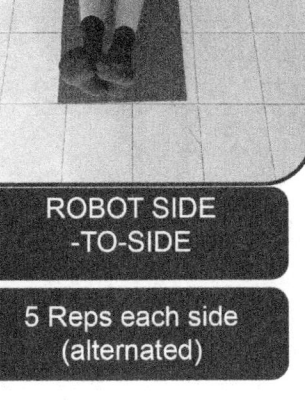

ROBOT SIDE -TO-SIDE

5 Reps each side (alternated)

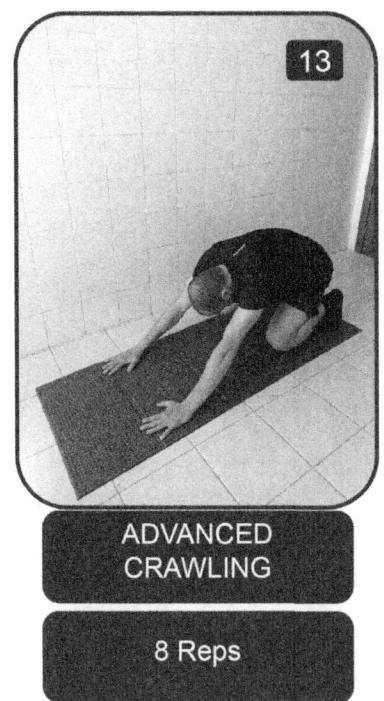

ADVANCED CRAWLING

8 Reps

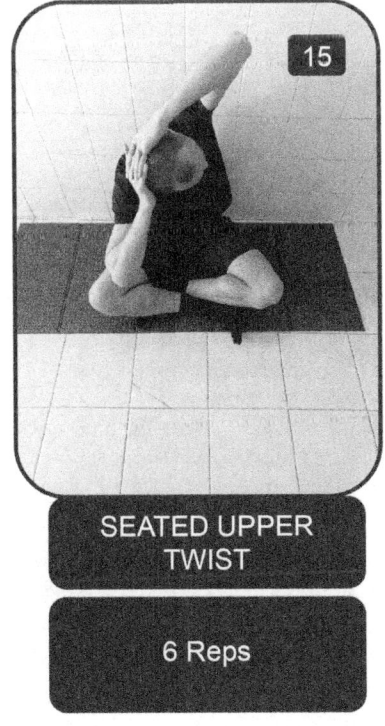

SEATED UPPER TWIST

6 Reps

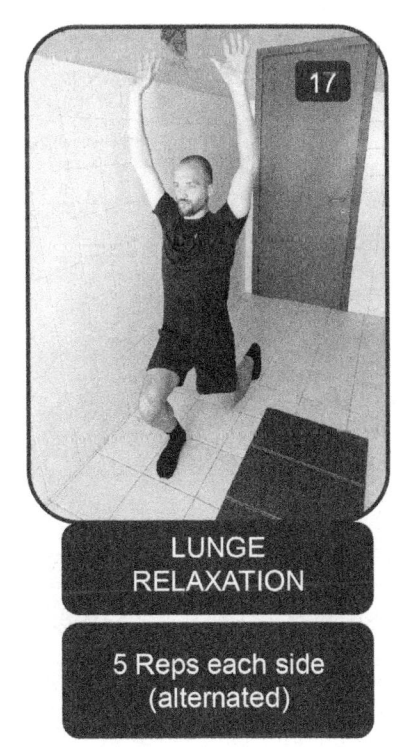

LUNGE RELAXATION

5 Reps each side (alternated)

Day 9 - Repeat it three times.

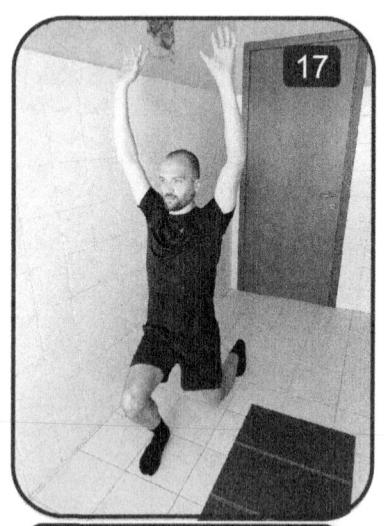

LUNGE RELAXATION

6 Reps each side (alternated)

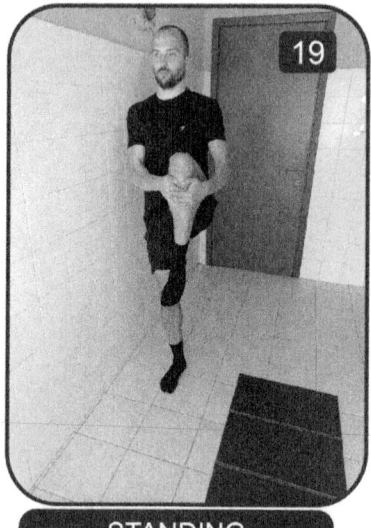

STANDING KNEE UP

6 Reps each side (alternated)

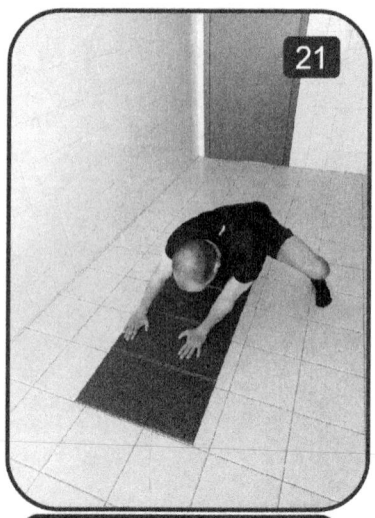

ADVANCED BODY CIRCLES

6 Reps each side

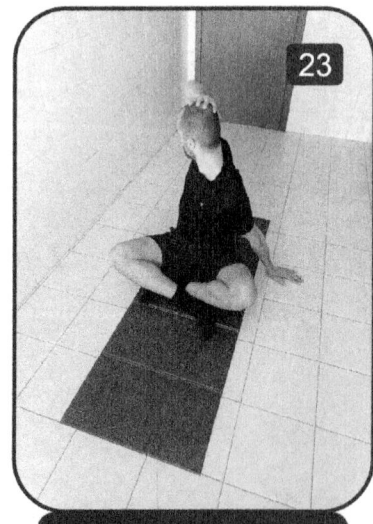

DIAGONAL OPENED TWIST

6 Reps each side

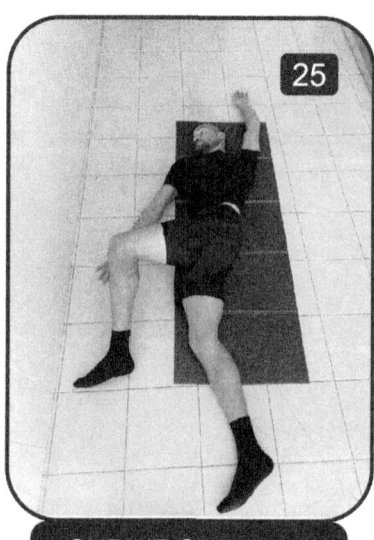

SUPINE STRETCH AND TWIST

3 Reps each side (alternated)

Day 10 - Repeat it three times.

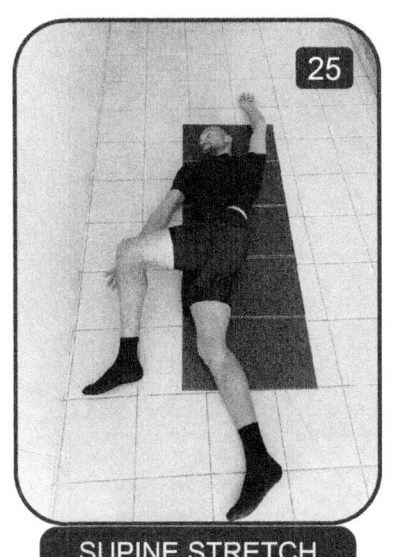

SUPINE STRETCH AND TWIST

4 Reps each side (alternated)

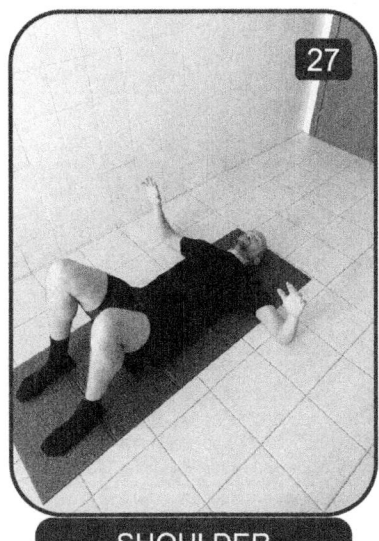

SHOULDER OPENING

6 Reps

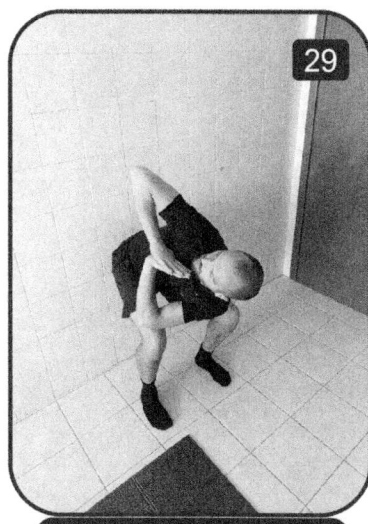

SEATED CHAIR TWIST

8 Reps each side (alternated)

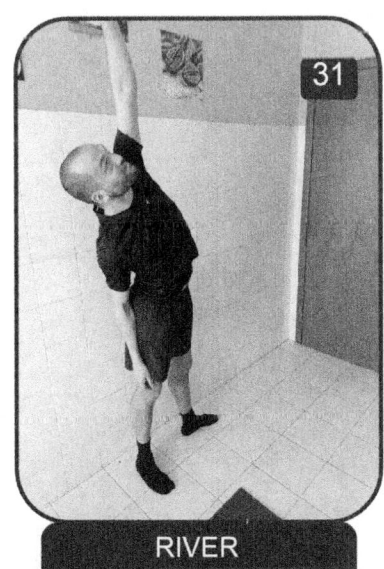

RIVER STRETCH

5 Reps each side (alternated)

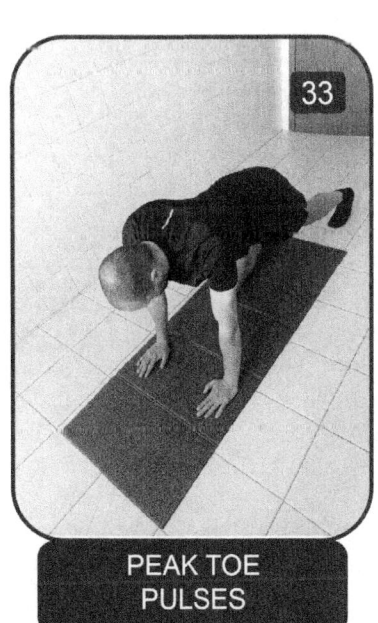

PEAK TOE PULSES

30 Seconds each side

Day 11 - Repeat it three times.

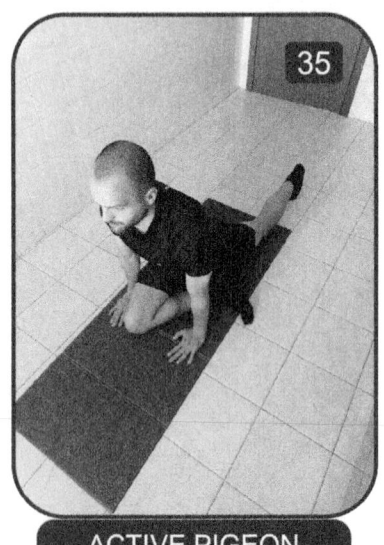

ACTIVE PIGEON STRETCH

5 Reps each side (alternated)

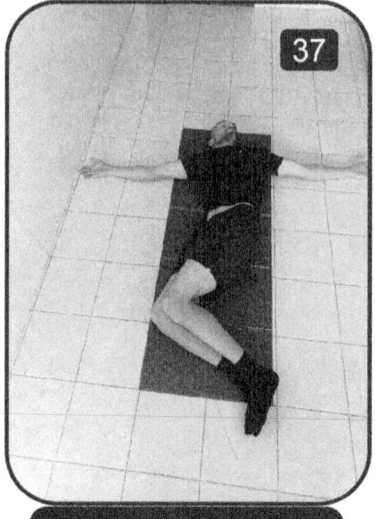

SIDE CHEST STRETCH

5 Reps each side (alternated)

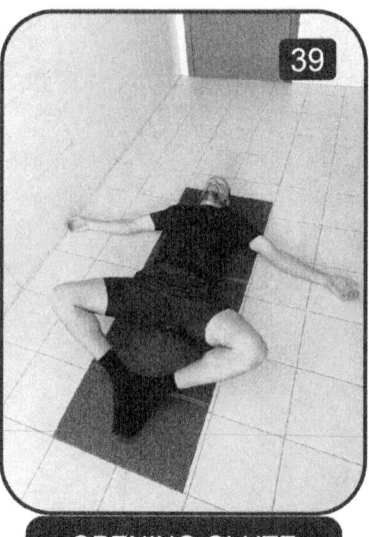

OPENING GLUTE BRIDGE

6 Reps

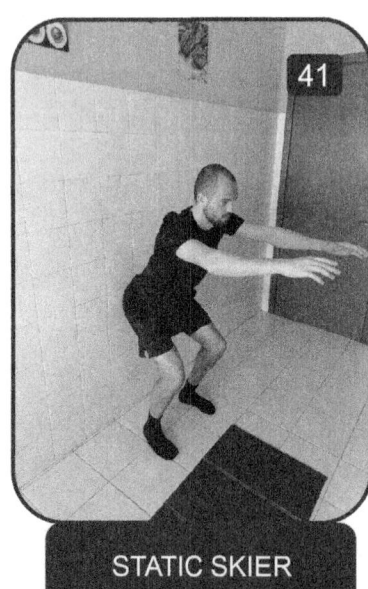

STATIC SKIER

30 Seconds

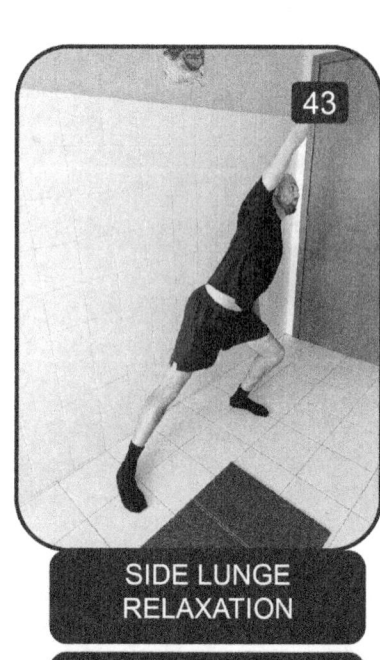

SIDE LUNGE RELAXATION

5 Reps each side (alternated)

Day 12 - Repeat it twice.

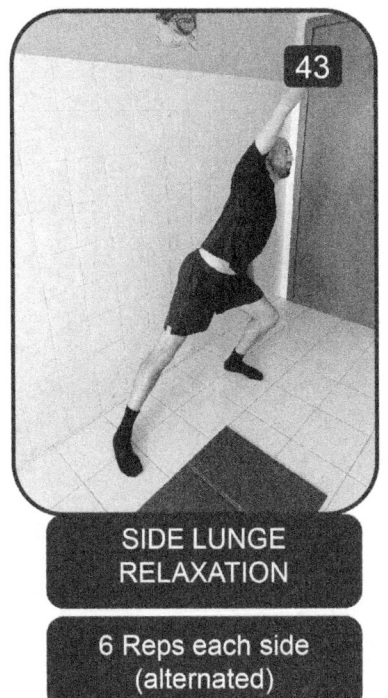

SIDE LUNGE RELAXATION

6 Reps each side (alternated)

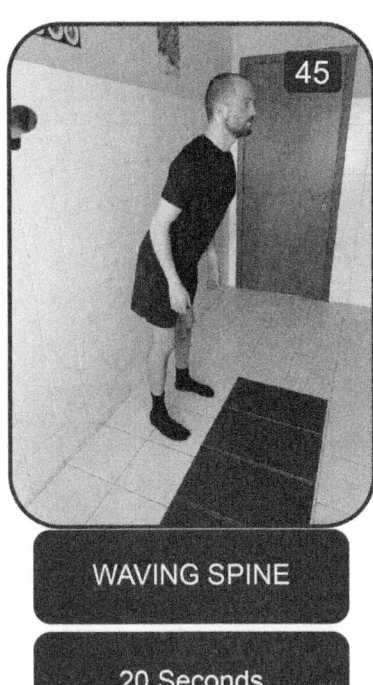

WAVING SPINE

20 Seconds

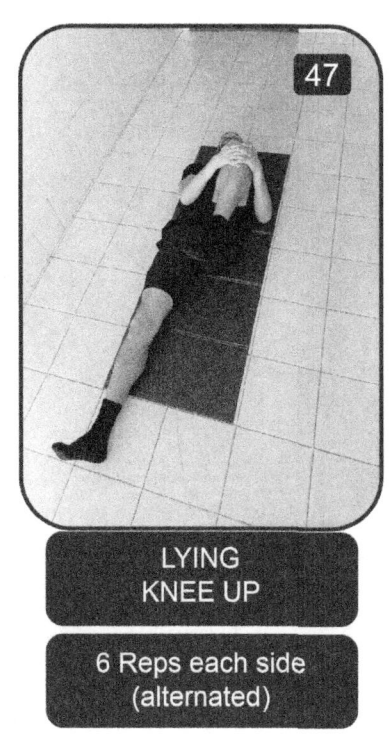

LYING KNEE UP

6 Reps each side (alternated)

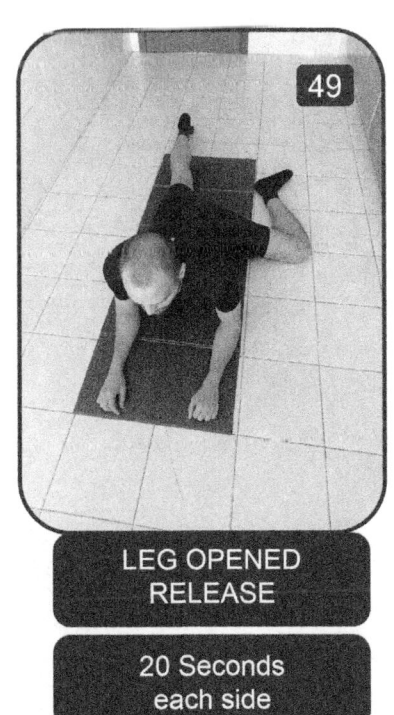

LEG OPENED RELEASE

20 Seconds each side

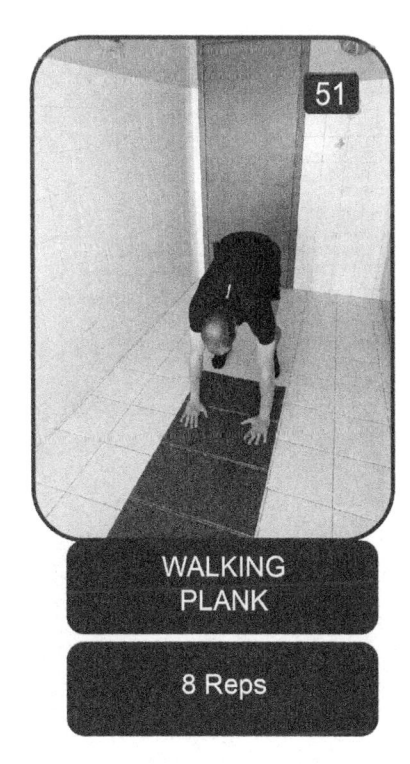

WALKING PLANK

8 Reps

Day 13 - Repeat it three times.

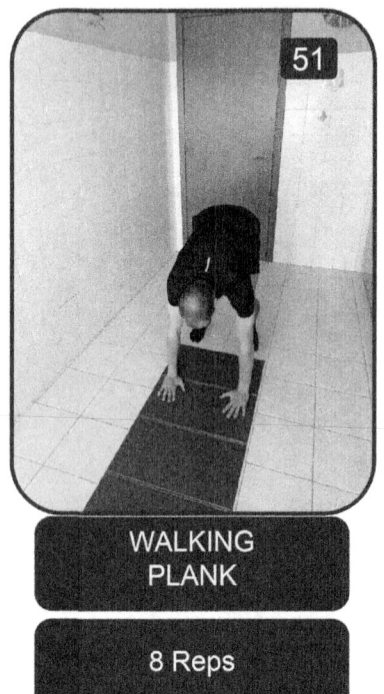

WALKING PLANK

8 Reps

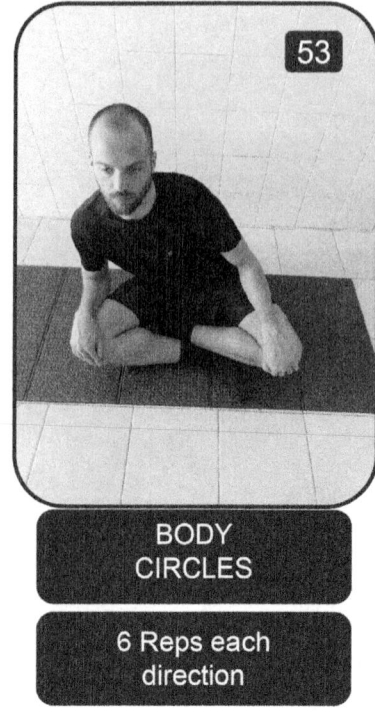

BODY CIRCLES

6 Reps each direction

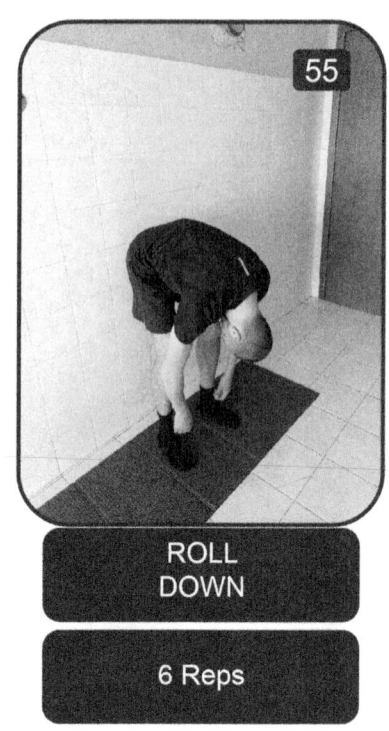

ROLL DOWN

6 Reps

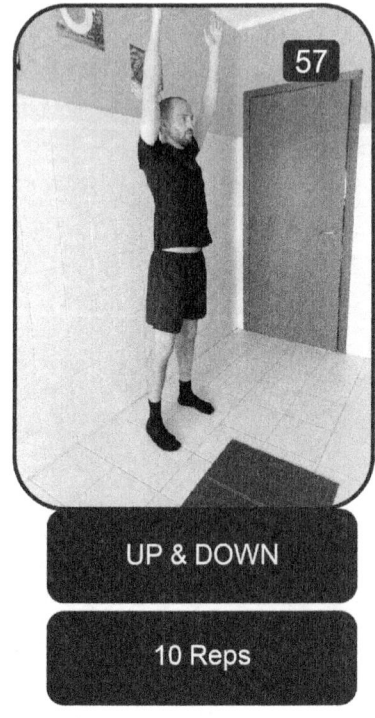

UP & DOWN

10 Reps

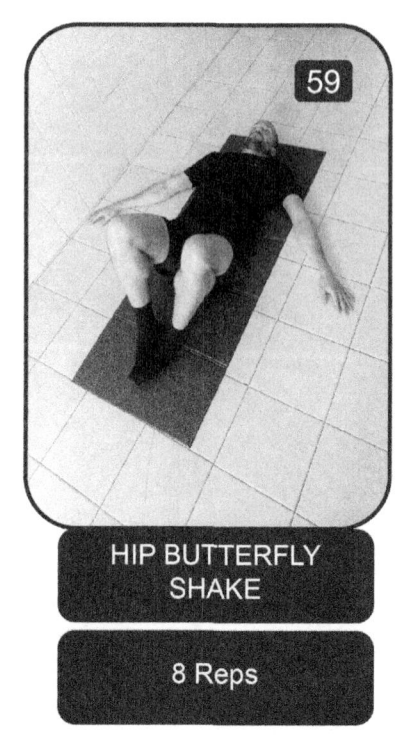

HIP BUTTERFLY SHAKE

8 Reps

Day 14 - Repeat it twice.

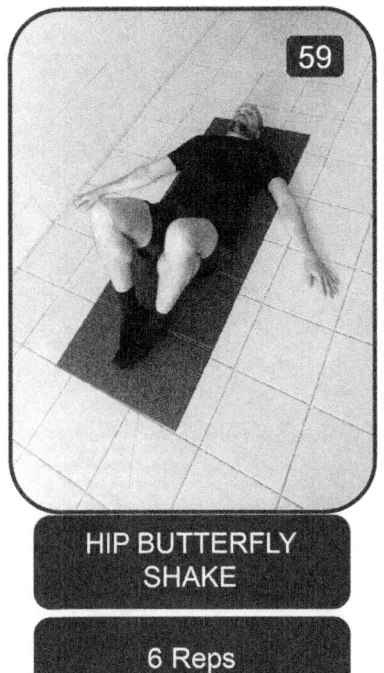

HIP BUTTERFLY SHAKE

6 Reps

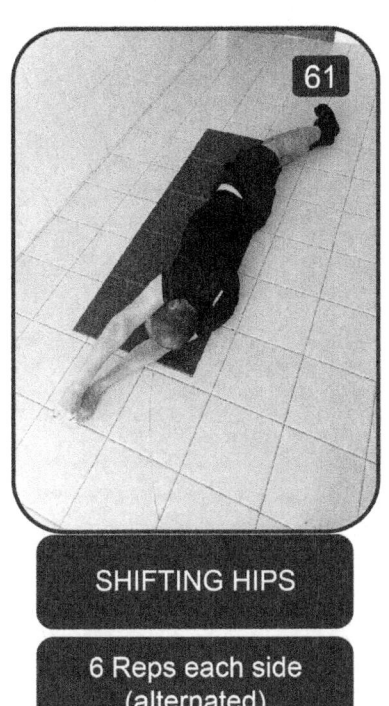

SHIFTING HIPS

6 Reps each side (alternated)

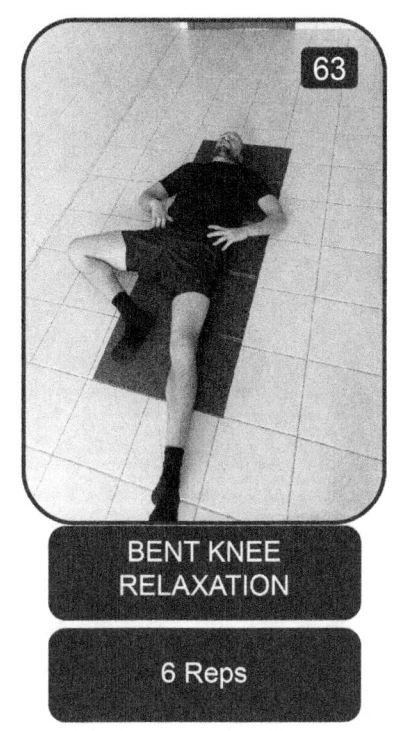

BENT KNEE RELAXATION

6 Reps

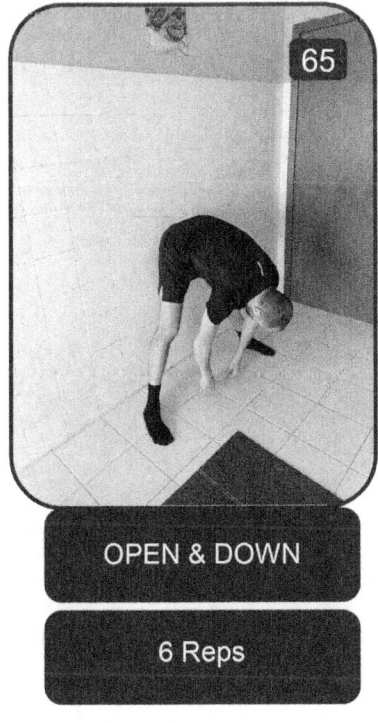

OPEN & DOWN

6 Reps

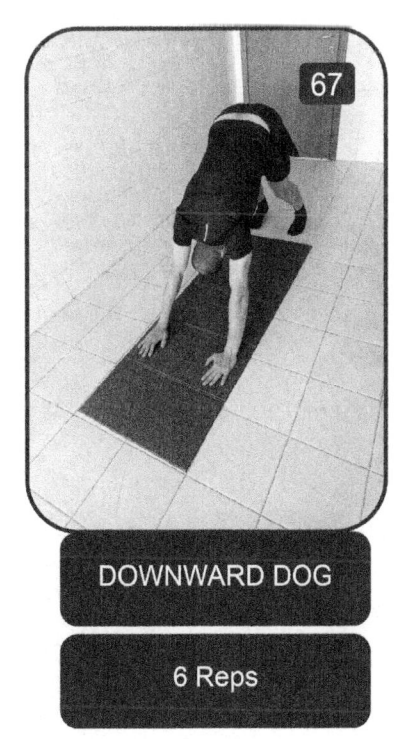

DOWNWARD DOG

6 Reps

Day 15 - Repeat it three times.

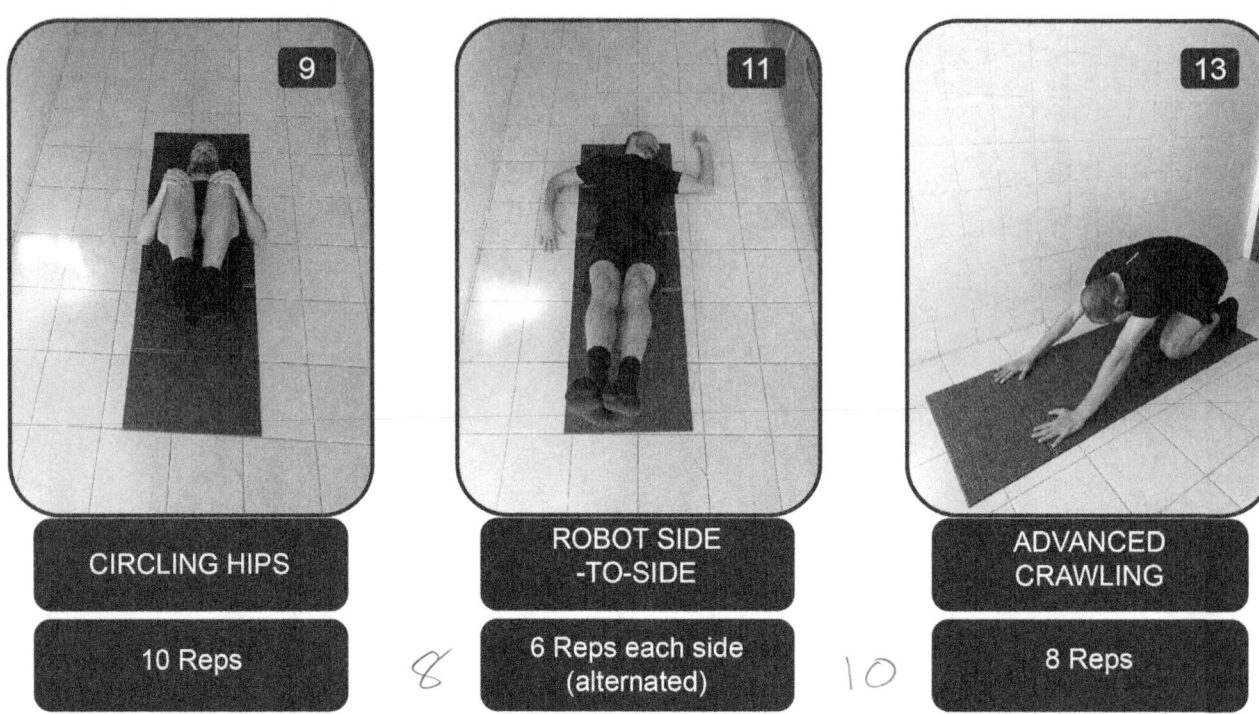

9	11	13
CIRCLING HIPS	**ROBOT SIDE-TO-SIDE**	**ADVANCED CRAWLING**
10 Reps	6 Reps each side (alternated)	8 Reps
14	8	10

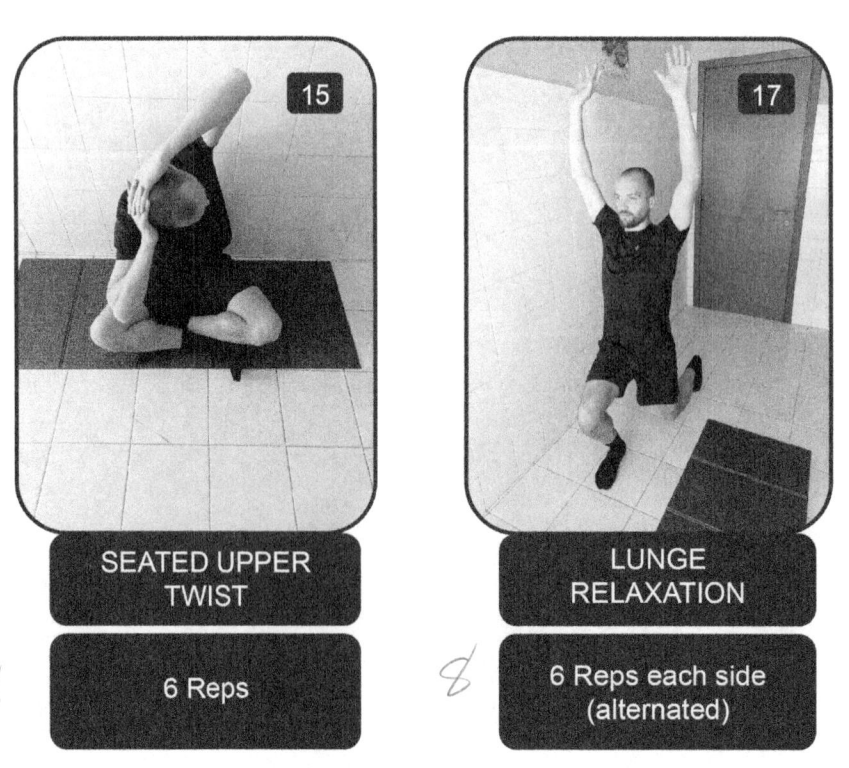

15	17
SEATED UPPER TWIST	**LUNGE RELAXATION**
6 Reps	6 Reps each side (alternated)
8	8

Day 18 - Repeat it three times.

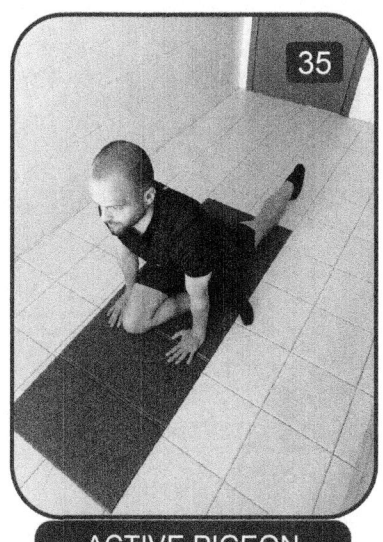

ACTIVE PIGEON STRETCH

5 Reps each side (alternated)

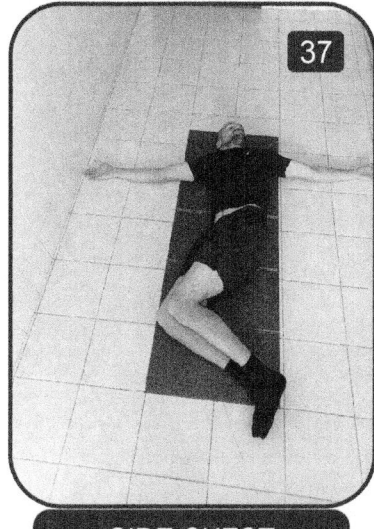

SIDE CHEST STRETCH

6 Reps each side (alternated)

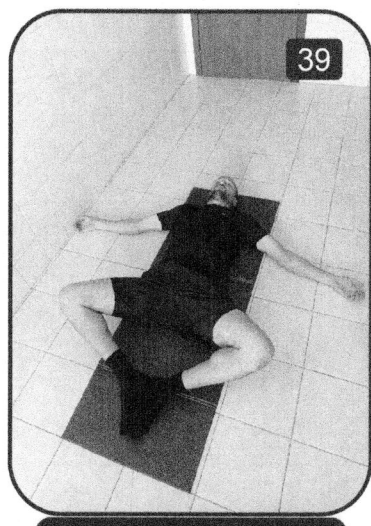

OPENING GLUTE BRIDGE

8 Reps

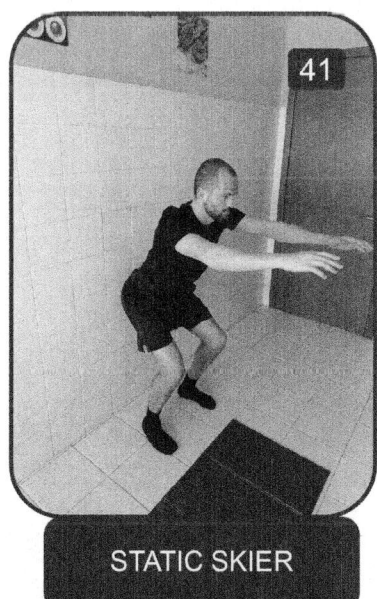

STATIC SKIER

30 Seconds

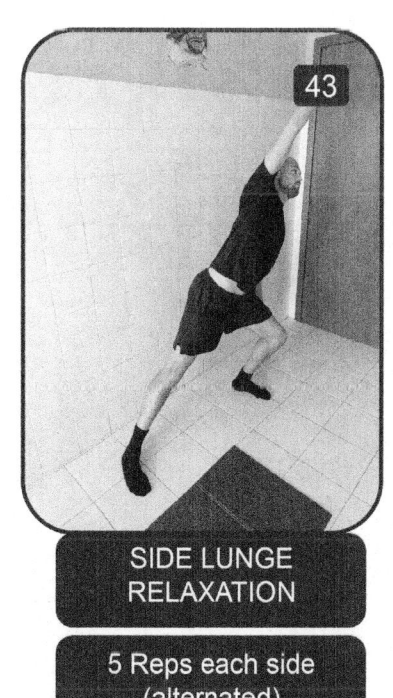

SIDE LUNGE RELAXATION

5 Reps each side (alternated)

Day 18 - Repeat it three times.

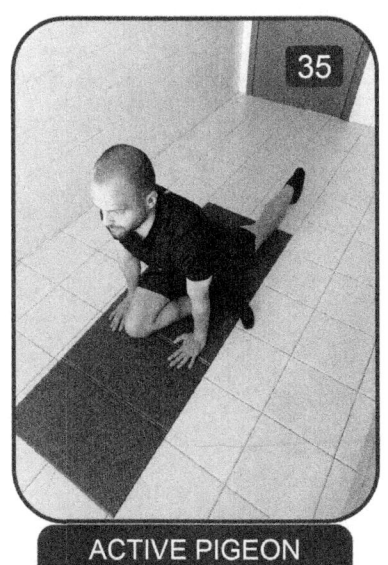

ACTIVE PIGEON STRETCH

5 Reps each side (alternated)

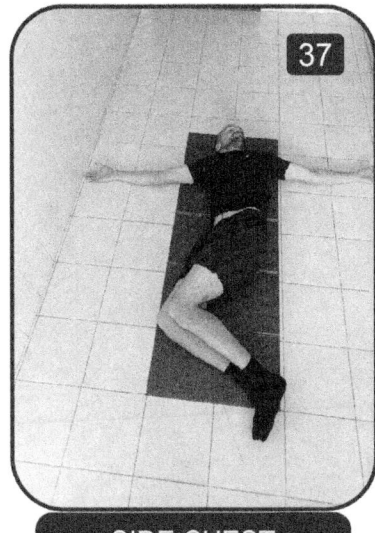

SIDE CHEST STRETCH

6 Reps each side (alternated)

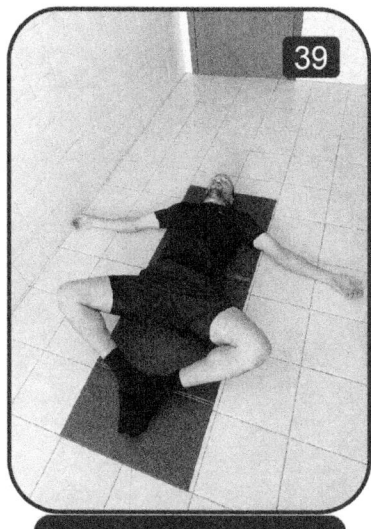

OPENING GLUTE BRIDGE

8 Reps

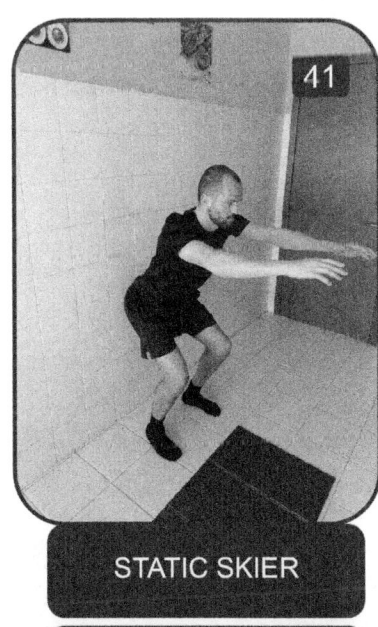

STATIC SKIER

30 Seconds

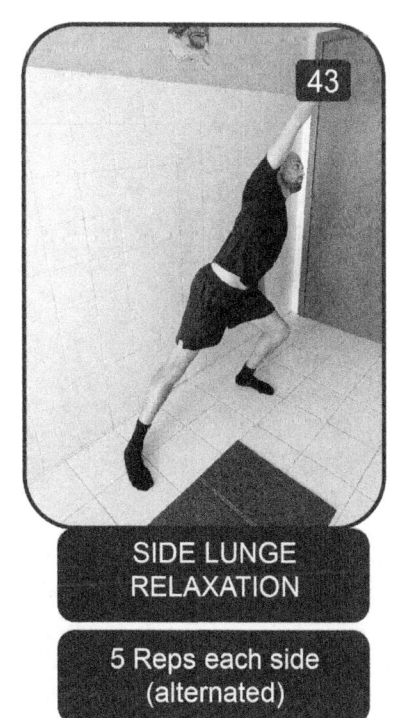

SIDE LUNGE RELAXATION

5 Reps each side (alternated)

Day 19 - Repeat it three times.

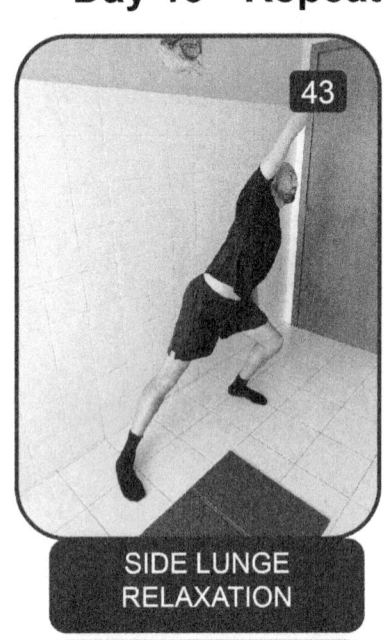

SIDE LUNGE RELAXATION

6 Reps each side (alternated)

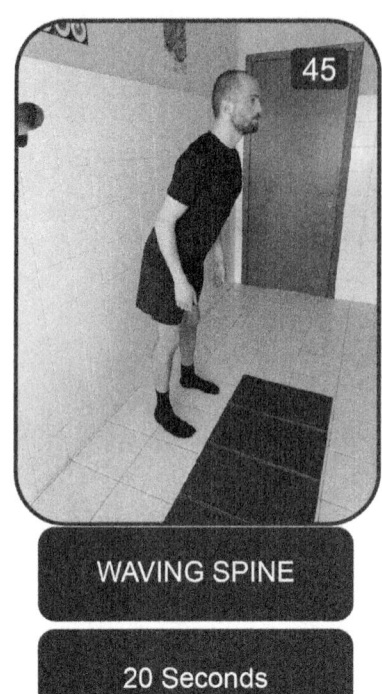

WAVING SPINE

20 Seconds

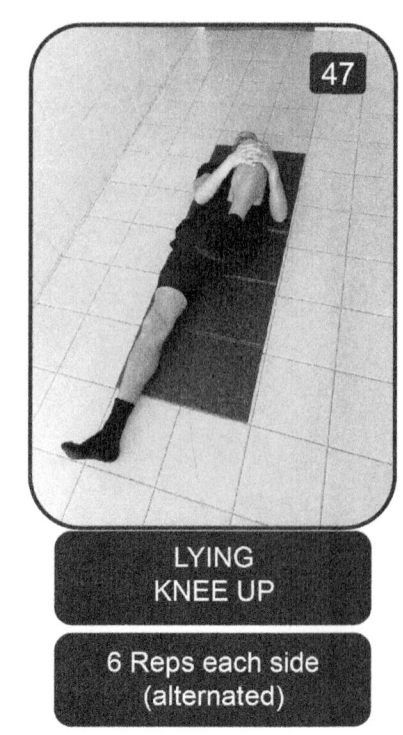

LYING KNEE UP

6 Reps each side (alternated)

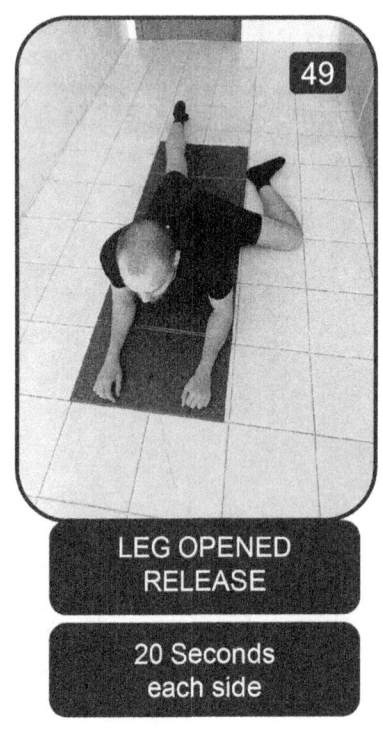

LEG OPENED RELEASE

20 Seconds each side

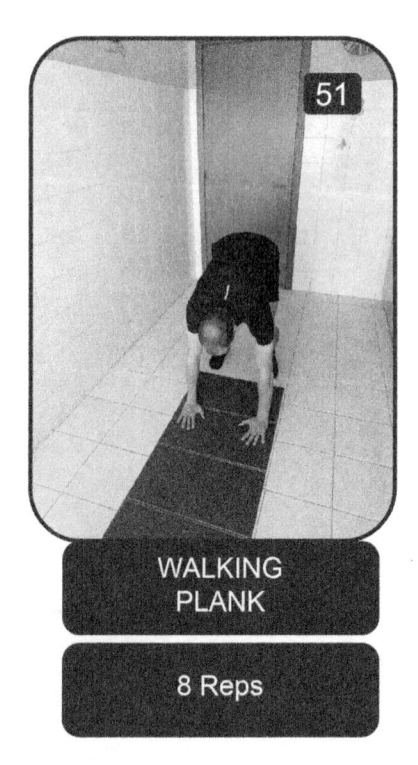

WALKING PLANK

8 Reps

Day 20 - Repeat it three times.

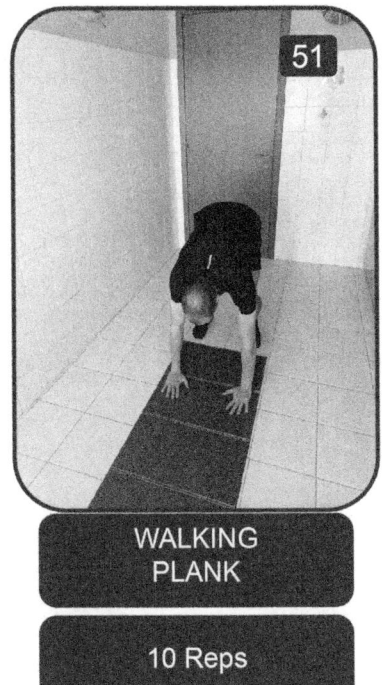

WALKING PLANK

10 Reps

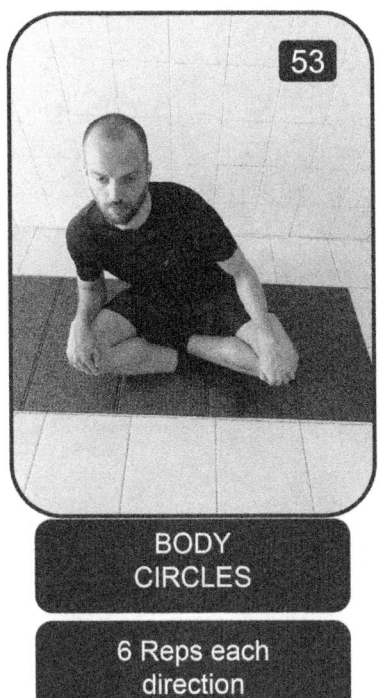

BODY CIRCLES

6 Reps each direction

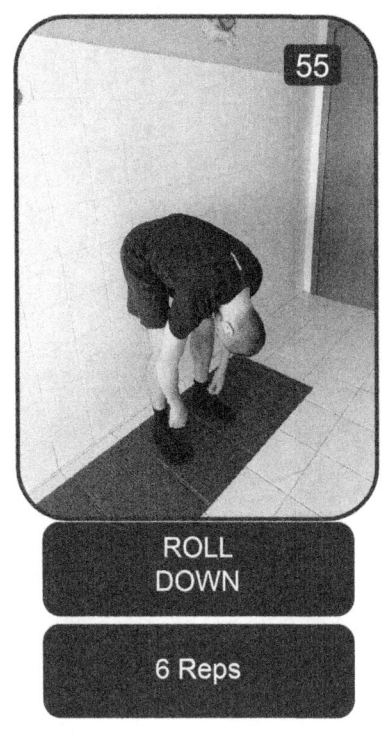

ROLL DOWN

6 Reps

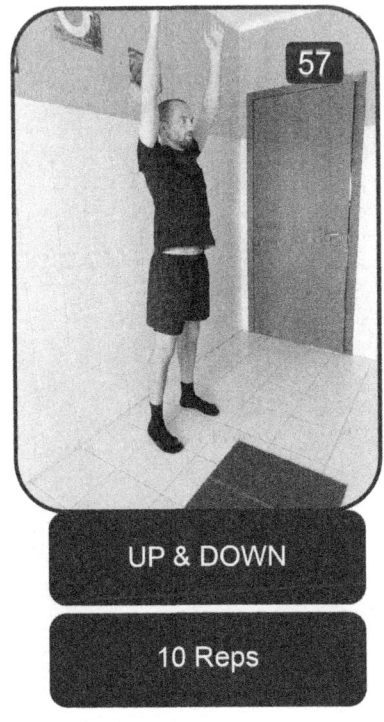

UP & DOWN

10 Reps

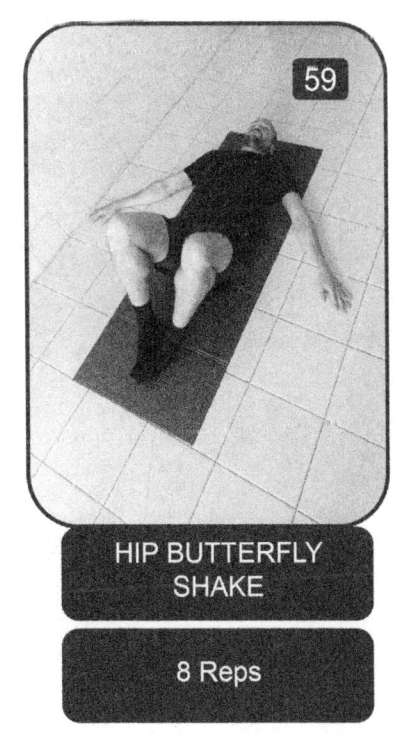

HIP BUTTERFLY SHAKE

8 Reps

Day 21 - Repeat it three times.

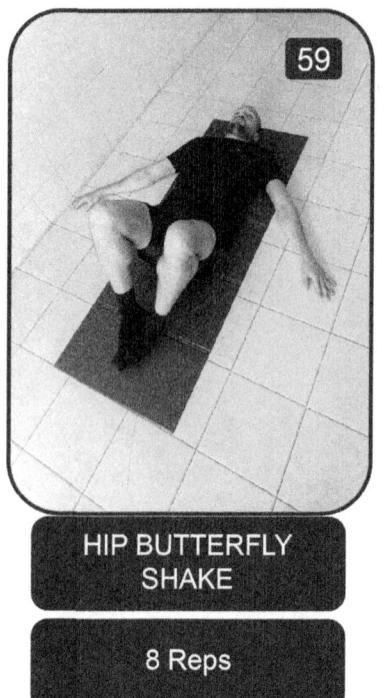

HIP BUTTERFLY SHAKE

8 Reps

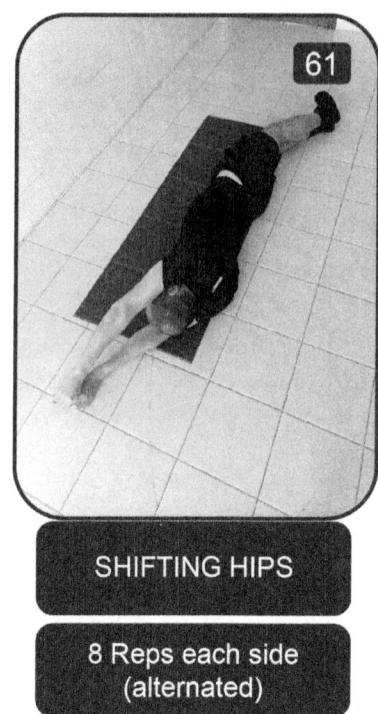

SHIFTING HIPS

8 Reps each side (alternated)

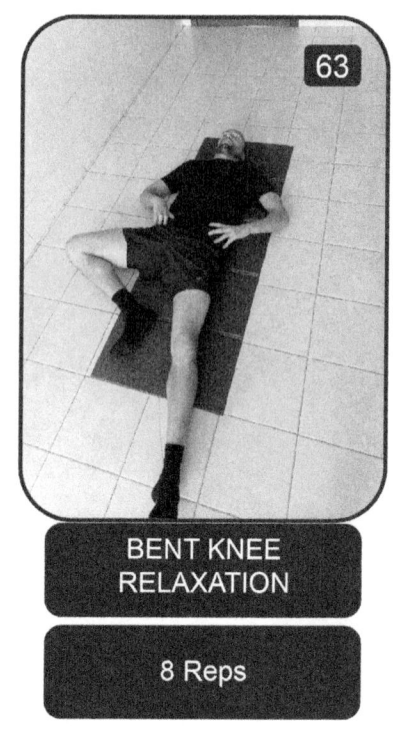

BENT KNEE RELAXATION

8 Reps

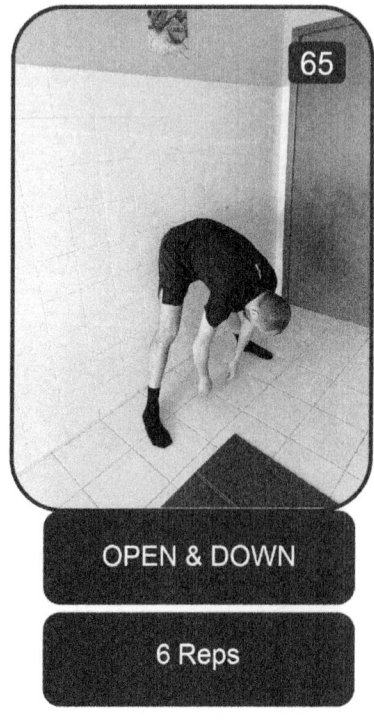

OPEN & DOWN

6 Reps

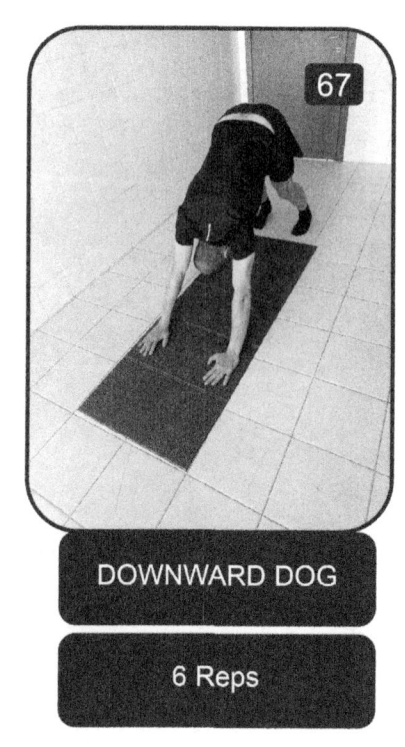

DOWNWARD DOG

6 Reps

Day 22 - Repeat it three times.

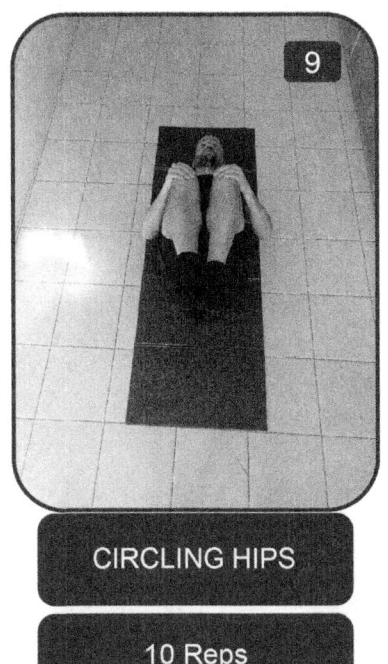

CIRCLING HIPS

10 Reps

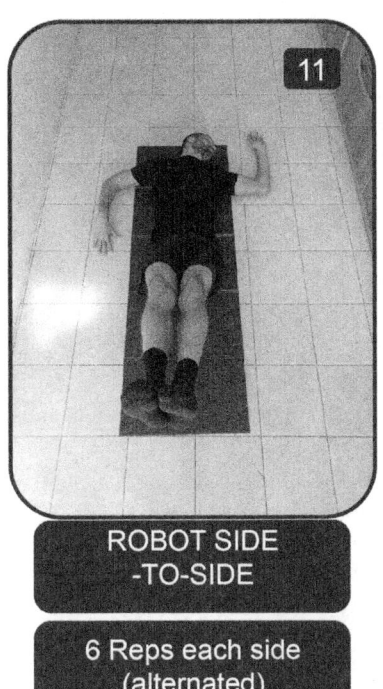

ROBOT SIDE -TO-SIDE

6 Reps each side (alternated)

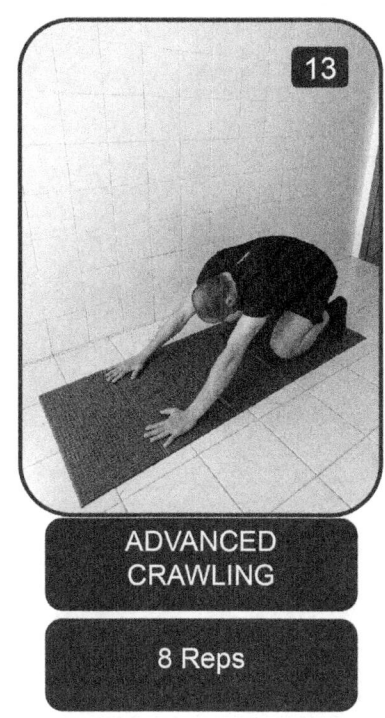

ADVANCED CRAWLING

8 Reps

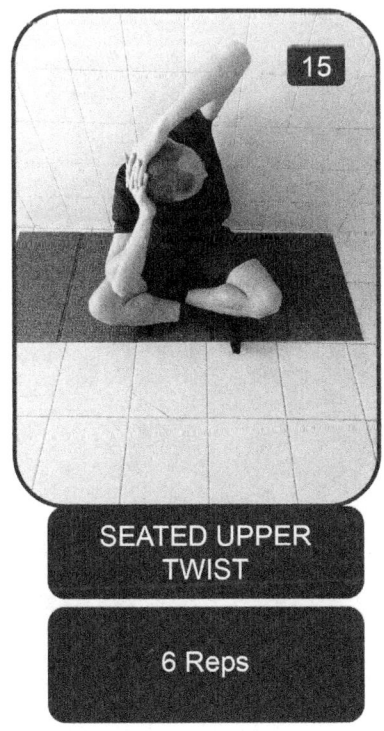

SEATED UPPER TWIST

6 Reps

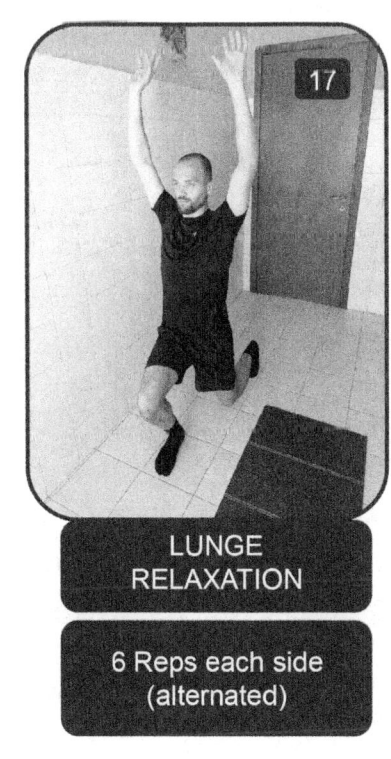

LUNGE RELAXATION

6 Reps each side (alternated)

Day 23 - Repeat it four times.

3

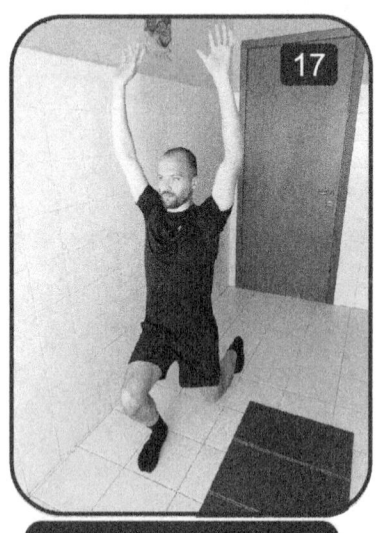

LUNGE RELAXATION

8

6 Reps each side (alternated)

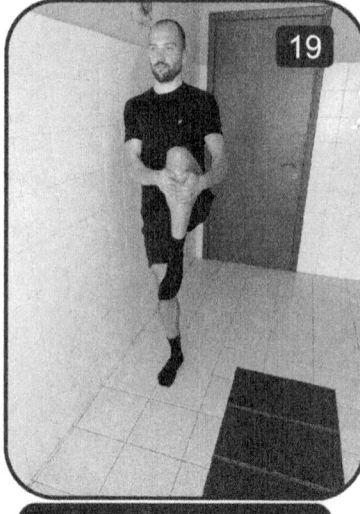

STANDING KNEE UP

8

6 Reps each side (alternated)

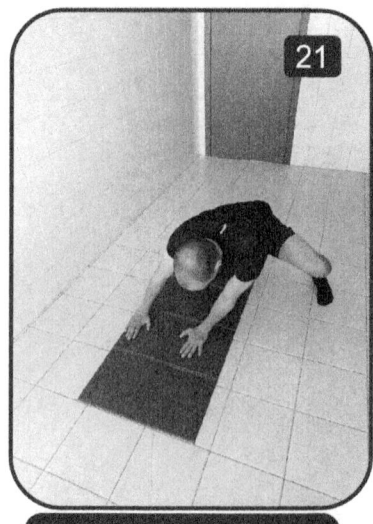

ADVANCED BODY CIRCLES

10

8 Reps each side

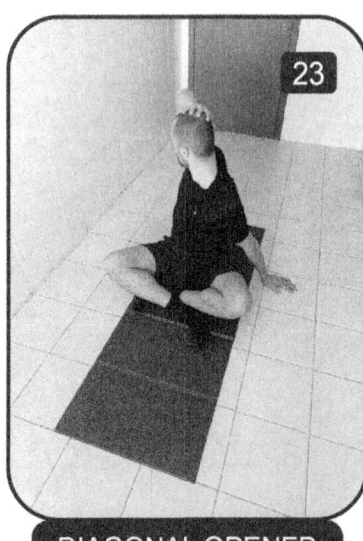

DIAGONAL OPENED TWIST

10

8 Reps each side

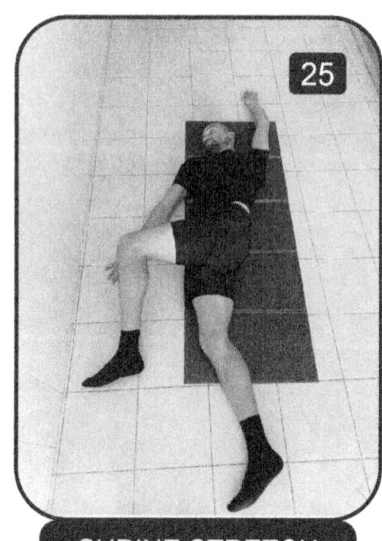

SUPINE STRETCH AND TWIST

4

3 Reps each side (alternated)

Day 24 - Repeat it three times.

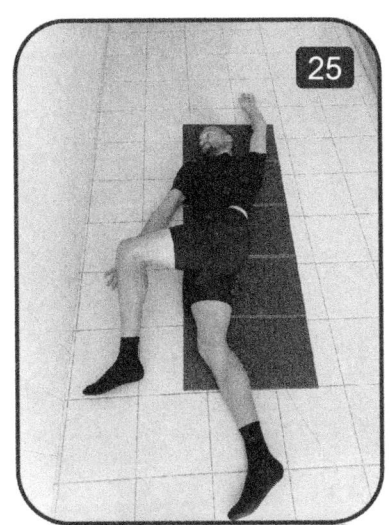

SUPINE STRETCH AND TWIST

4 Reps each side (alternated)

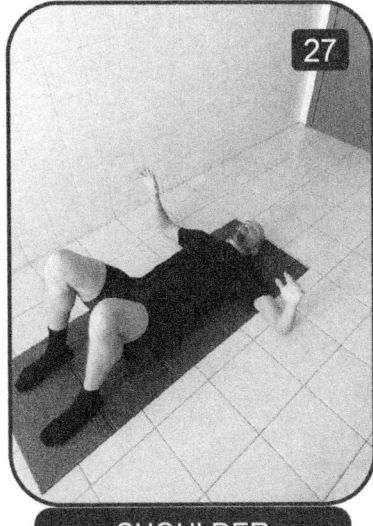

SHOULDER OPENING

8 Reps

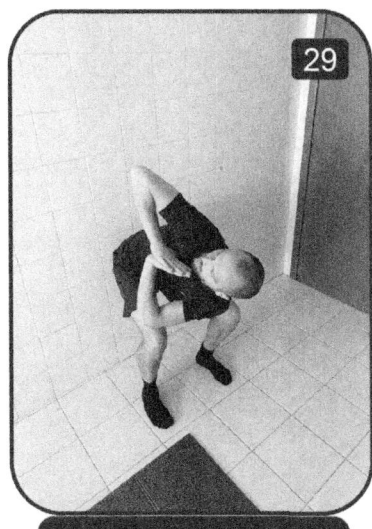

SEATED CHAIR TWIST

8 Reps each side (alternated)

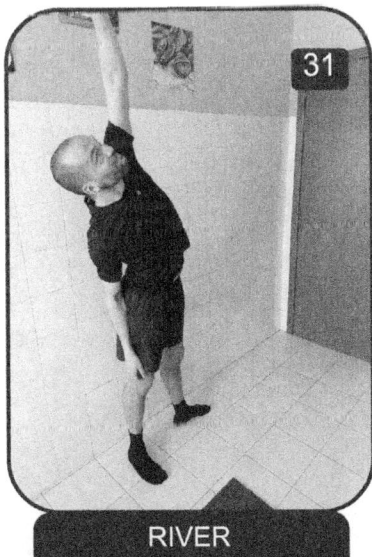

RIVER STRETCH

8 Reps each side (alternated)

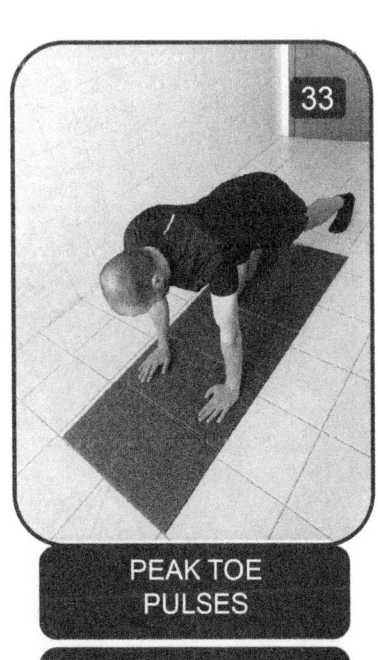

PEAK TOE PULSES

30 Seconds each side

Day 25 - Repeat it four times.

3

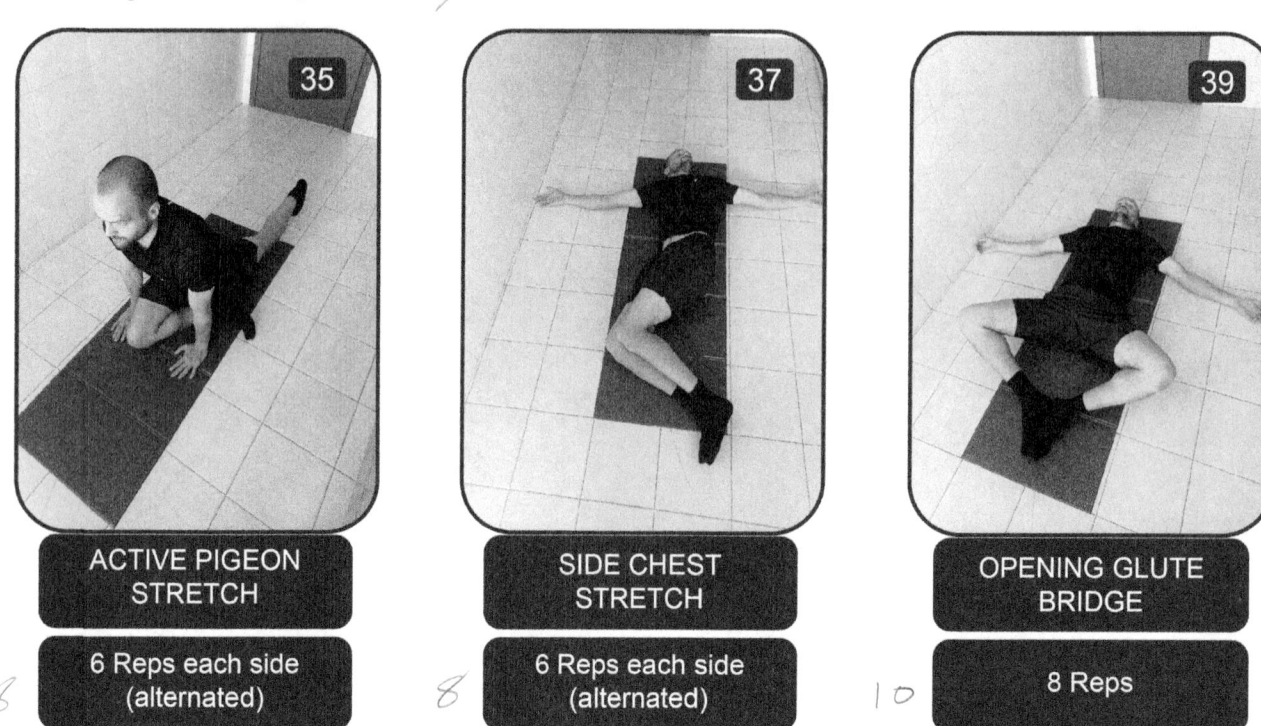

35	37	39
ACTIVE PIGEON STRETCH	**SIDE CHEST STRETCH**	**OPENING GLUTE BRIDGE**
6 Reps each side (alternated)	6 Reps each side (alternated)	8 Reps

8   8   10

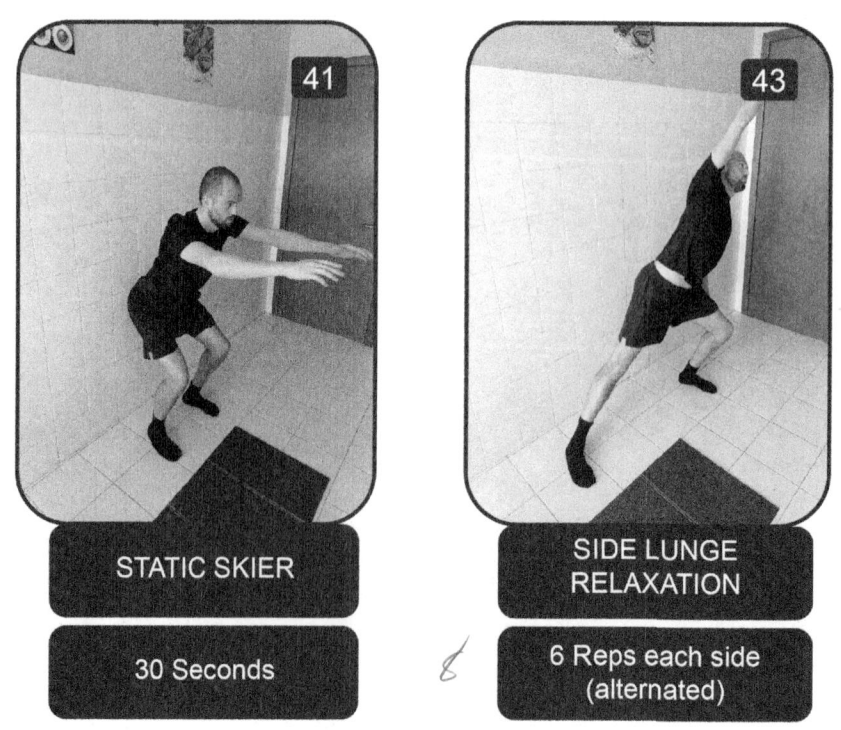

41	43
STATIC SKIER	**SIDE LUNGE RELAXATION**
30 Seconds	6 Reps each side (alternated)

40   8

Day 26 - Repeat it three times.

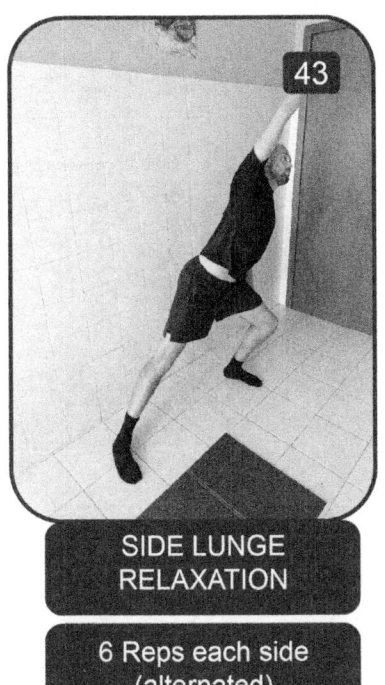

SIDE LUNGE RELAXATION

6 Reps each side (alternated)

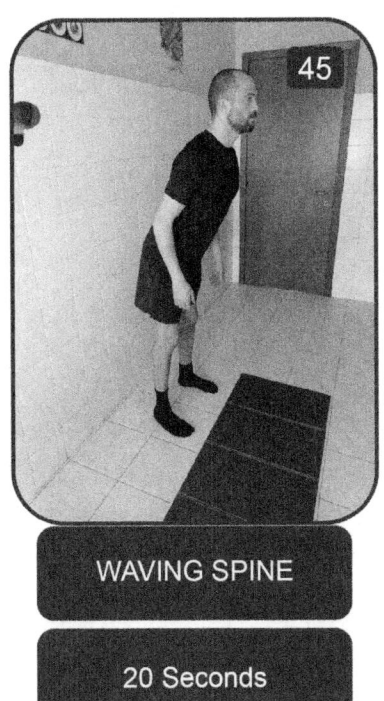

WAVING SPINE

20 Seconds

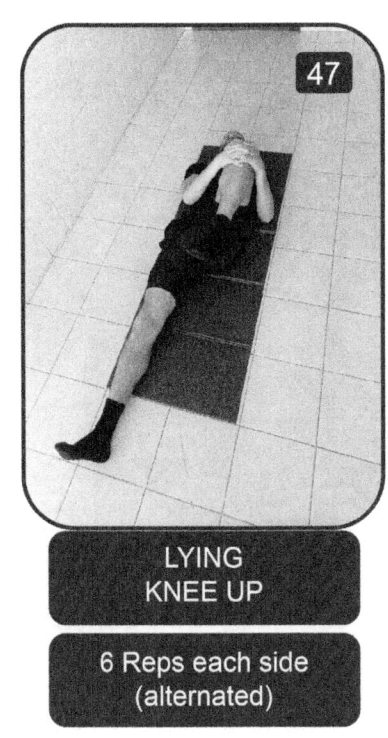

LYING KNEE UP

6 Reps each side (alternated)

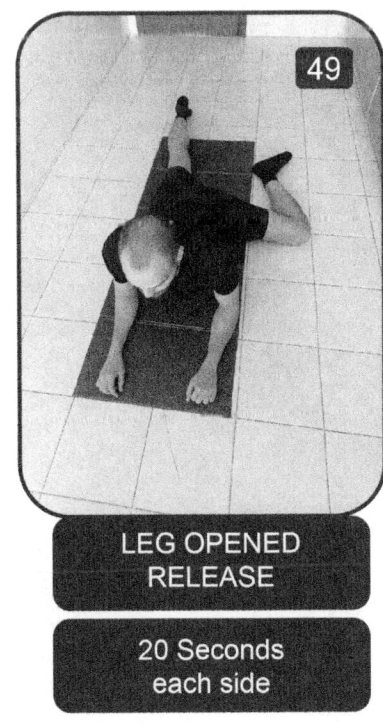

LEG OPENED RELEASE

20 Seconds each side

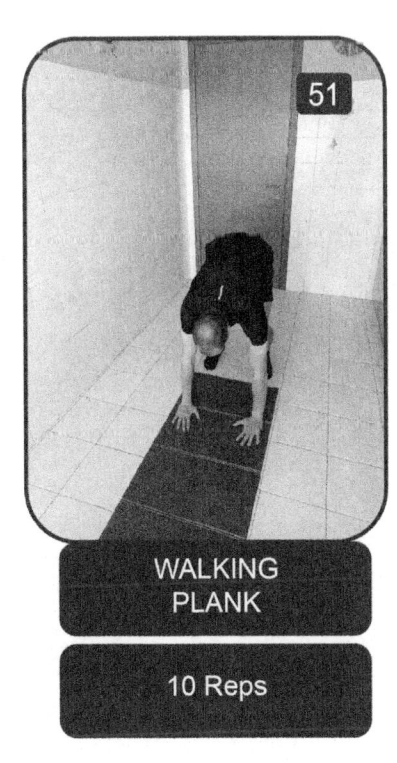

WALKING PLANK

10 Reps

Day 27 - Repeat it four times.

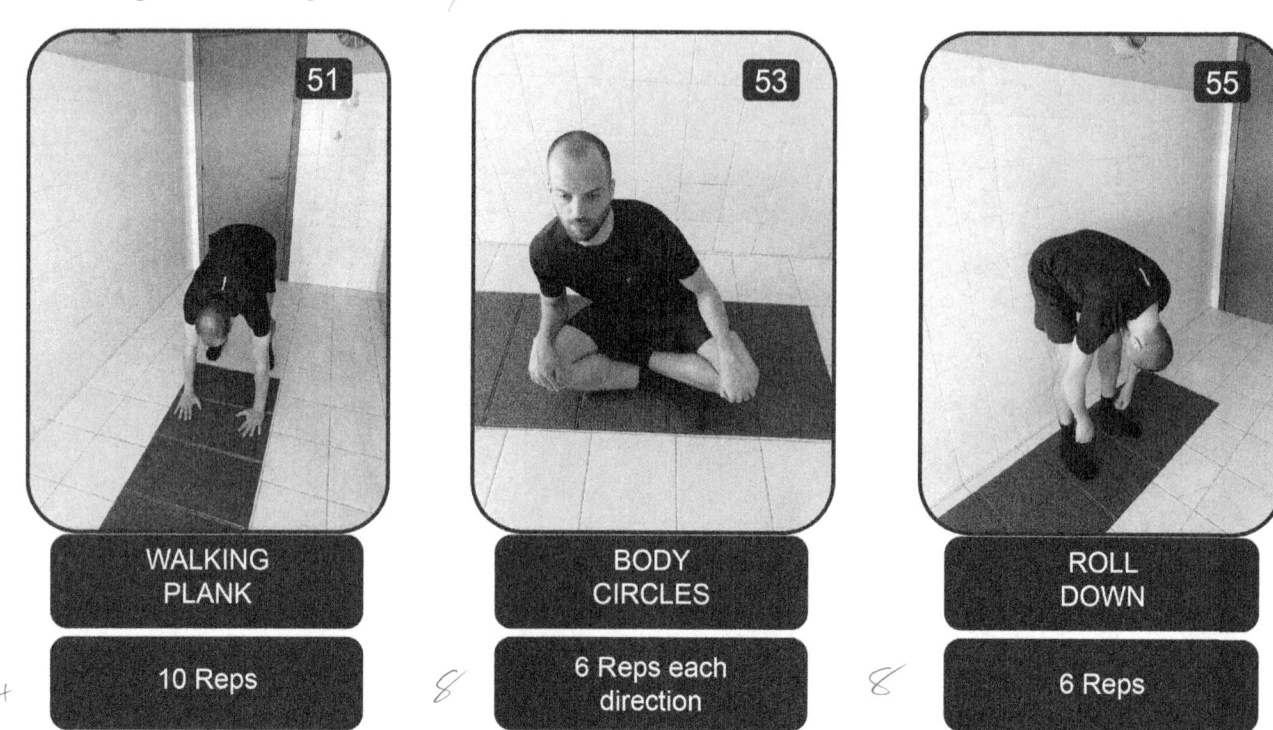

51 WALKING PLANK — 10 Reps	**53** BODY CIRCLES — 6 Reps each direction

55 ROLL DOWN — 6 Reps

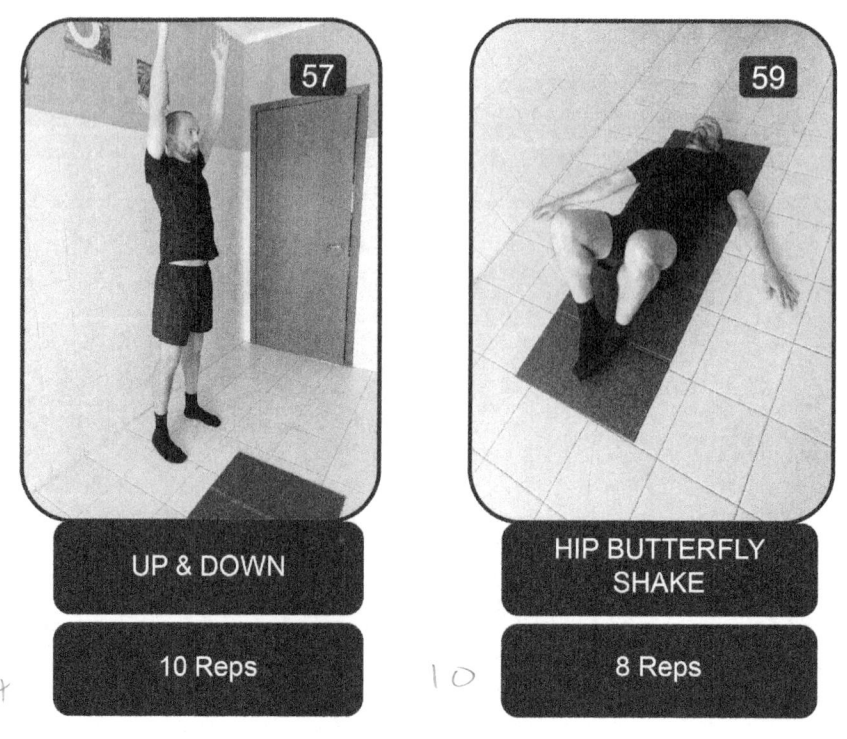

57 UP & DOWN — 10 Reps

59 HIP BUTTERFLY SHAKE — 8 Reps

Day 28 - Repeat it three times.

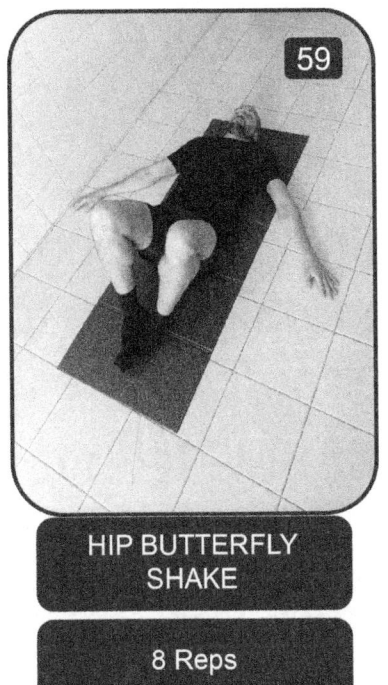

HIP BUTTERFLY SHAKE

8 Reps

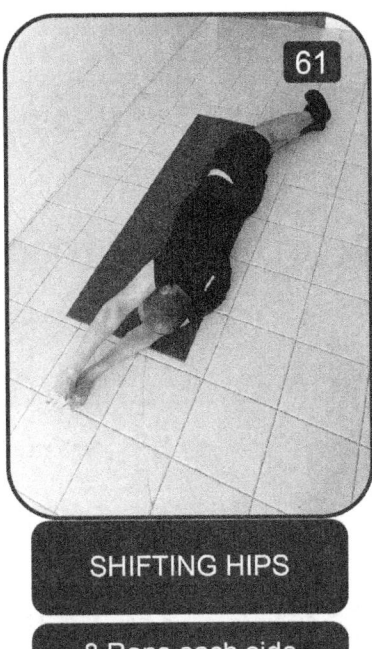

SHIFTING HIPS

8 Reps each side (alternated)

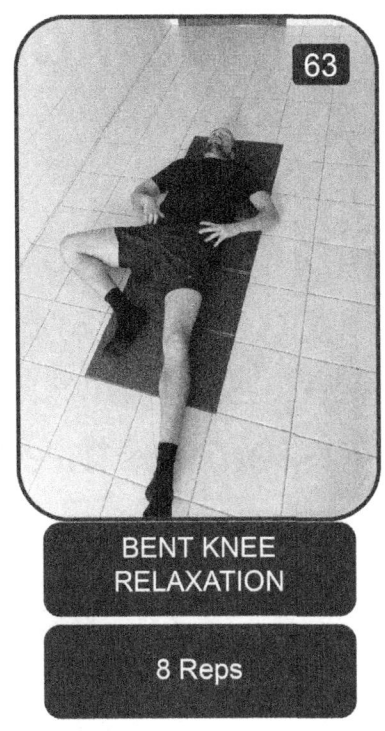

BENT KNEE RELAXATION

8 Reps

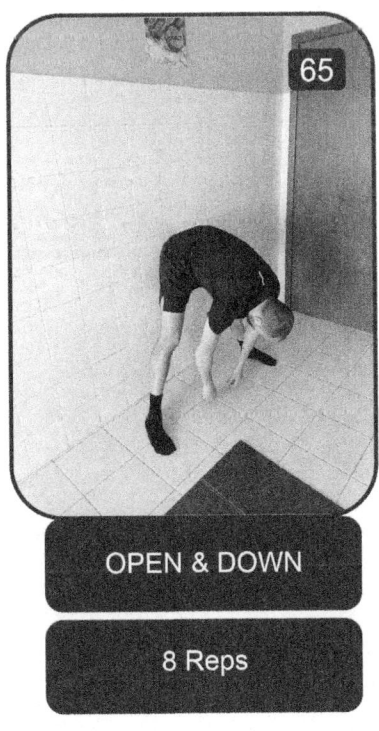

OPEN & DOWN

8 Reps

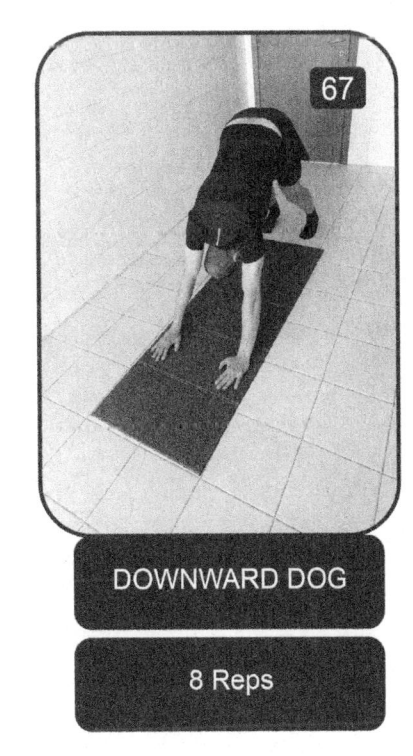

DOWNWARD DOG

8 Reps

Well done for finishing these 28-days!

I suggest you take 3 days off from training (although long walks are fine), and then resume from day 15 to day 28. For each workout, aim for four or five sets instead of three or four (add one set for each day).

For any questions or doubts feel free to email me at somatictrainingplan@gmail.com

CONCLUSION

Congratulations on finishing the book! I hope you enjoyed reading it. I really wanted this book to help you learn a lot, give you new exercises, and show you how special somatic practices can be.

I believe that every exercise in this book can help you live a happier and healthier life. These exercises have various benefits for your body and mind and can help you let go of stress and tough feelings that you might feel.

I'm sending you my best wishes for lots of happiness and success in the next few months. I hope this book will be a good guide for you as you work on being healthier and stronger. I hope the exercises make you happy and give you strength as you face new challenges with courage.

If you have any questions or doubts, feel free to contact me at

somatictrainingplan@gmail.com, and I'll be happy to assist you the

best I can about somatic exercises and workouts!

Printed in Great Britain
by Amazon

46328730R00057